LIVE
WELL

LIVE WELL

100 simple ways
to add years to your life

Dr. Trisha Macnair

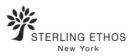
STERLING ETHOS
New York

CONTENTS

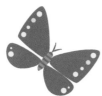

INTRODUCTION

Life today has much to offer, and simply thinking positively about your own well-being helps you to live a healthier life. The more of that "feel-good" factor you have, the better you are likely to do at work, for example, and the more money you are likely to earn, so you can buy healthier food, afford to go to the gym and take relaxing vacations. You are also more likely to work better in a team and get on well with others. Contented people make more friends and have better relationships—all things that can contribute to a greater feeling of wellness.

We are wealthier than ever before, with more time and money to spend on what we really enjoy, yet we can still struggle to identify how these resources can be best used to improve our lives. We need to actively play a part by adopting a lifestyle that promotes general well-being.

While you can't change factors like your genetic make-up, you can begin to understand their effects on your physical well-being and how they could affect your future. The moment you are conceived, you are dealt a certain set of cards for life. Those cards—your genes—will have a myriad of powerful influences on how well

and how long you live. Equally, other influences are handed down in childhood: a healthy diet in childhood may protect against disease later in life. Cultural views on the roles of men and women, for example, also influence longevity. How your parents or grandparents taught you to behave—whether smoking was acceptable, or whether vaccination was considered the devil's magic—may stay with you for life.

Your genes aren't totally in charge of your body, and this book suggests many ways in which you can take wellness back into your own hands. After all, you have a choice about many aspects of the way you live your life, from what you eat to how you exercise. Studies of twins—a standard way of looking at the influence of our genes—show that only about 25 percent of the variation is the result of inherited factors. That means that the greatest influence by far on the length and quality of your life is what happens to you during your lifetime.

Live Well contains a wealth of little, easy to follow ideas to help you take control of your well-being, and make the most of all that life has to offer.

BE CONSCIENTIOUS

Conscientiousness has been shown to be associated with a longer, healthier life. The Terman Life-Cycle Study, which ran from 1922 to 1991, found that adults who weren't very conscientious during their childhood died at a younger age.

Conscientiousness is related to emotional intelligence and involves being thoughtful, thorough, organized, and committed. It can make a person more aware of their own health needs, and more likely to take a serious view of the prevention of disease. This characteristic also tends to be visible in harder-working and more reliable individuals. For instance, conscientious people are more likely to get vaccinated or have regular physical exams and screening tests, exercise even when they don't feel like it, eat healthy foods when they would really rather eat a bar of chocolate and avoid risk-taking activities such as drinking, drugs, and dangerous sports.

Being conscientious may also develop into care for others and the community, which builds stability and support in your own life as well as in the lives of others. A conscientious person is also more likely to react constructively to challenges, and is more likely to create work and living environments that promote good health.

LOVE A PET

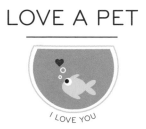

I LOVE YOU

All you need is love, and even the love of a goldfish might do. Having a pet that you can talk to and interact with may add to the quality of your life.

Studies have found that petting or being near a familiar animal can lower heart rates and blood pressure levels. One US study looked at male and female stockbrokers already taking medication to control high blood pressure. Those with pets had significantly lower heart rate and blood pressure levels, which didn't become so raised when they were asked to do mental arithmetic and other stressful tests. This was particularly marked when the pet was nearby during the stressful event, when there was just half the increase in blood pressure compared with participants who did not own a pet.

Another New York study, conducted by Allen, Blascovich and Mendes in 2002, reported that, after suffering a heart attack, those people who owned a dog were six times more likely to be alive one year later than those who didn't. People with pets visit their doctors less, and are less likely to suffer from depression.

A pet may bring you new friends, too. People find companionship and comfort not just from the pets themselves, but also because they are more likely to engage with others through owning the animal.

KEEP MOVING

Arthritis means inflammation of the joints, bones, and supporting tissue. There are more than 100 types but most common by far is osteoarthritis. If you looked closely at people over 60 you would find almost every single one had some degree of osteoarthritis. Osteoarthritis has a profound effect on health expectancy, causing chronic pain and reduced mobility, interfering with a person's ability to exercise, disturbing their sleep patterns, and seriously reducing quality of life. Other types of arthritis such as rheumatoid arthritis—where, in addition to joint problems, one may suffer severe inflammation of other tissues, including the heart—may more directly impinge on longevity, as well as quality of life.

How to reduce the risks of osteoarthritis

- Reduce excess weight so that your joints don't have to bear large loads.
- Do regular gentle exercise to help build up the strength, stability, and range of motion of your joints. But you should avoid doing high-impact exercise such as aerobics, which can put excessive strain on the joints.
- If you have osteoarthritis, ask your doctor about drug treatments such as nonsteroidal anti-inflammatory drugs that help to minimize joint damage. When the disease is more severe, aim to maintain mobility using drug treatments or, if it becomes necessary, surgery (joint replacements, for example).

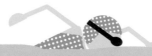

4

BELIEVE IN YOURSELF

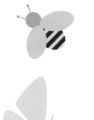

Confidence has a direct impact on mental and physical well-being. Some psychologists believe that confidence is a more powerful determinant of success than innate ability. It can make us more or less vulnerable to stress and depression, and it influences how far we are likely to persevere in the face of difficulties. It affects the immune system and activates endorphins, our natural painkillers.

Self-confidence is a set of beliefs about yourself, not an inherent skill or personality trait. You can be very competent and capable and still feel a lack of self-confidence, but it is possible to improve your confidence level, and it is worth trying to do so. Do this by focusing on the positives in your life. Recognize what you are good at and try to implement those things more into your daily routine.

KEEP A FOOD JOURNAL

Food journaling, particularly if you're on a diet, is a useful way to see what and how much you really eat. But beyond that, food journaling can give you accurate insight into how you eat emotionally and how the food you eat affects your body.

- By recording and quantifying every item of food that passes between your lips, you make yourself more accountable for your diet.
- You may be motivated to make better decisions because you can actually see where your calories are coming from and how nutritional your choices are.
- Note how you are feeling before, during, and after your meal, so you can pinpoint your emotional triggers and actively work to counter any negative habits.
- A food journal is also a useful tool for tracking food allergies. Scribble down any reactions you have to your food, and patterns may arise that you can talk about with your doctor.

Use a journal platform that works for you and your busy life, whether that is a notebook that you can carry around in your handbag or an app on your phone. At first you may find it difficult to maintain a food journal, but once you get used to recording your meals, you will find that they lead you to a greater understanding of your food and your body.

6

SAY HIGH TO FIBER

HELLO FIBER!

Fiber is particularly recommended as a protection against cardiovascular disease and cancer, but tests involving a high-fiber diet have produced varying results, either suggesting an insignificant reduction in death from any cause, including heart disease, or proposing a 28 percent reduction in the likelihood of developing heart failure.

The case against cancer is stronger, however, as animal experiments show a reduction in colon cancer. Surveys of people who eat a lot of fiber suggest that this works for humans, too, although trials where fiber has been specifically added to the diet to prevent cancer haven't shown an effect. Meanwhile, one study has shown that fiber from cereals and fruit may protect against breast cancer.

Although the real value of this much-lauded element of our diet isn't clear, it's best, for now, to keep going for the grain: A long-term, high-fiber diet will increase your well-being, even if it doesn't add years to your life.

How to add necessary fiber to your diet

- Eat soluble fiber found in legumes, fruit, and vegetables. It lowers cholesterol levels, helps delay absorption of foods, and aids blood sugar control.
- Eat insoluble fiber, from wholegrain cereals, fruit and vegetables, as it improves bowel function.

7

SPEND TIME IN NATURE

"Better beans and bacon in peace than cakes and ale in fear", says the country mouse in Aesop's fable. The town mouse had scoffed at his country cousin's basic diet and taken him to feast in the town. But, chased by large dogs and stressed by urban living, the country mouse soon retreated home.

Both urban and rural life have advantages for health but in general, the more urbanized a nation, the higher the average life expectancy. Development of cities and towns tends to reflect industry, wealth, good communications, and an established social support system. However, within many cities there are areas of intense deprivation where segregated groups live in substandard housing while battling typical urban problems such as traffic pollution and a lack of green space.

So although living in an urbanized nation may help you to live longer, it may be better, if you can afford it, to choose the more rural areas within that nation. If you have to live in a town or city, having walkable green space nearby—and using it—has been shown to be associated with living well for longer.

ESCAPE URBAN POLLUTION

It's a frightening prospect to think that the air you breathe could be killing you, but research has shown that living in heavily industrialized areas can affect life expectancy because of pollution in the air.

Polluting particles are released into the atmosphere when wood and fossil fuels are burned—clouds of them are emitted from the exhaust pipes of vehicles, for example. They can also form in the air from mixtures of pollutant gases. Larger particles fall quickly to the ground but fine particles stay in the air for much longer and can be carried by the wind long distances from their emission sources.

The World Health Organization has warned that a large number of health problems result from exposure to fine particles, which pass into the lungs when inhaled. Respiratory and cardiovascular diseases can develop or be aggravated by particle pollution.

So pack your bags for the countryside—or, better still, start lobbying your government representative!

GET VACCINATED

Adults are often vulnerable to the same infectious threats children are—no matter what your age, vaccination will help you to live a longer life. The side effects of vaccinations are generally minimal and major problems very rare—they are certainly rarer than the risk from the disease you are being vaccinated against.

If you haven't already had the standard childhood vaccines, talk to your doctor to see which ones you might need. Adults may be just as vulnerable to the effects of many of these infections; in fact, some of them cause a much more severe illness if caught in adult life.

Adults need a tetanus vaccination, for example, just as much as children do, and should have a booster dose every 10 years. This disease (also known as lockjaw) is found all over the world and may be fatal in up to 20 percent of cases. Gardeners should be particularly careful to keep their tetanus immunization up to date—tough, resistant spores of the bacteria that cause tetanus (*Clostridia*) are found in the soil, and enter the body through any wound or scratch that punctures the skin.

People who travel frequently also need to make sure they are fully vaccinated against the infections that pose a risk in the country they are visiting.

ADULTS ARE OFTEN VULNERABLE TO THE SAME INFECTIOUS THREATS CHILDREN ARE. NO MATTER WHAT YOUR AGE, VACCINATION WILL HELP YOU TO LIVE A LONGER LIFE.

New vaccines may dramatically affect life expectancy in the future. A vaccine that offers protection against human papilloma viruses (HPV, the cause of cancer of the cervix and other genital cancers) is now available, and many other anti-cancer vaccines are in the pipeline.

Child immunizations

An immunization program from two months to 13 years might include:

- Diphtheria.
- Tetanus.
- Whooping cough (acellular pertussis).
- Measles and Mumps.
- Polio.
- Influenza.
- Hemophilus influenzae type b (Hib).
- Rubella (German Measles).
- Meningitis C.
- Hepatitis A and B.
- Pneumococcal conjugate (PCV13).
- Tuberculosis.
- Chickenpox.

EMBRACE SIBLING RIVALRY

If you have lots of brothers and sisters, you probably know what it can be like to grow up in a large family, fighting for attention and competing with one another to get enough food at the dinner table. You might think you're missing out on the tranquility and one-on-one attention a single child enjoys.

Think again—as you get older, the "protective role" of the large family kicks in, and the benefits of having plenty of people around begin to show. Research has found that grandparents who have few siblings live shorter lives than those with lots of siblings. If you're a parent, you'll notice a similar effect from having lots of children: They might wear you out when you are a young parent, but in the end they help to keep you going.

So, whether you're an only child or from a big family, surround yourself with friends and family to enhance your quality of life—and theirs.

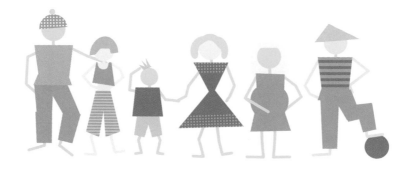

HAVE A LITTLE FAITH

In virtually every one of more than a thousand studies examining the effects of spirituality on healing, a powerful link was found between faith and longevity. A 12-year study at the University of Iowa found that those who attended religious services at least once a week were 35 percent more likely to live longer than those who never attended a church or other faith-based events.

Being actively involved in a spiritual community—by going to religious services regularly, for example—boosts the immune system and helps to keep high blood pressure and clogged arteries at bay. It is associated with lower levels of Interleukin-6, a mediator of inflammation linked to age-related diseases such as atherosclerosis. Researchers speculate that this positive effect is the result of a healthier diet and lifestyle among churchgoers. The strong sense of community that most religions offer also plays a part.

LOOK AT THE VIEW

If you're lucky enough to live or work in a pleasing environment—surrounded by gentle gardens, for instance—you'll know how much this counts towards providing a deep sense of well-being every day. Unsurprisingly, research has shown that after an operation, those patients who were assigned to hospital rooms with a pleasant outdoor view (of trees, for example) recovered faster and were discharged sooner than those who had a view of a brick wall.

Now, if a good view helps patients recover, it must surely help the rest of us keep healthy by lifting our mood, easing stress and providing a deep sense of optimism and contentment. So park your chair by the window and take a good look outside. If you don't like what you see, put up posters or paint pictures on the wall—or just make sure you get out and spend some time every day somewhere where the view is good.

STRENGTHEN YOUR BONES

As you age, your bones become less dense, and their internal scaffolding breaks down. This process, known as osteoporosis, makes the bones fragile and susceptible to fracturing. It's a particular problem in women, where it results from the decline in levels of female hormones that occurs after menopause. It has been estimated that osteoporosis will affect 15 percent of women at the age of 50, 30 percent at 70 and 40 percent at 80. Combined with an increasing weakness of the muscles and the failing sense of balance that occurs with age, osteoporosis creates a recipe for disaster. Many cases of falls in the elderly result in a fractured or broken bone, often the hip or a vertebra. The consequent immobility leads to muscle wasting, loss of confidence, and an increased risk of infections such as pneumonia.

How to keep osteoporosis at bay

- Build up your bones by getting the recommended daily amounts of calcium (1,000–1,300 milligrams) and vitamin D (400–800 IU) from a young age.
- Take dietary supplements if necessary.
- Do weight-bearing exercise (such as walking, running, tennis, or dancing) several times a week.
- Avoid smoking and excessive alcohol.
- From about age 65 (age 60, if you are at an increased risk of osteoporosis), go for bone density tests and take medication recommended by your doctor.

EXERCISE REGULARLY

The effects of regular exercise on mental well-being alone could add as much as two or more years to your life. The Harvard Alumni Study, which took into account more than 71,000 men who had graduated from Harvard University and the University of Pennsylvania between 1916 and 1954, found that those men who regularly burned 2,000 calories a week while exercising lived, on average, two years longer than those who chose to live a sedentary life.

Exercise works its magic because it is good for almost every system in the body. Although most of its effects are on physical health, it also works wonders on the psyche. People who exercise several times a week, whether to a moderate or intense degree, have lower levels of stress, anger, anxiety, and depression.

The bonus is that once you experience greater mental well-being, you are even more likely to engage in physical activity. So drag yourself out of that couch-potato rut, and you'll find it gets even easier to exercise.

15

HAVE HEALTHY PARTNERS

The state of your health as you get older is influenced to a considerable degree by the health of your partner, as well as the rest of the family, so you'll want to make sure that you and your partner keep an eye on each other's health.

Illnesses can be transmitted between partners during close contact or simply while sharing the same environment. Many infections, such as colds and mild gastroenteritis, are minor and short-lived. But others, such as meningitis, hepatitis, or HIV, can have a profound effect on health and life expectancy.

Among elderly couples, the health of the "unit" (that is, both partners living together) may be essential in enabling them to support each other to live independently in their own home. It is often the case that when one of them becomes ill, the other struggles to cope without the mental and physical support of their partner, eventually becoming vulnerable to accidents and illness themselves.

Looking after your partner's health is all part of your own health agenda. Encourage your partner to follow the steps in this book, and make sure they seek help when things aren't right.

THE HEALTH OF THE "UNIT" IS ESSENTIAL IN ENABLING COUPLES TO SUPPORT EACH OTHER TO LIVE INDEPENDENTLY.

LOVE YOUR HEART

Disease of the heart and blood vessels (which together are known as cardiovascular disease) is the Number 1 killer in developed nations. Although statistics vary from country to country, cardiovascular disease causes serious problems for half the population of the western world, and is to blame for about one in three deaths. According to the American Heart Association, life expectancy would increase by at least seven years if all forms of cardiovascular disease were eliminated.

Coronary artery disease (where the blood vessels to the heart are clogged) causes chest pain, shortness of breath, and heart failure, and can result in a heart attack. Stroke (damage to the brain as a result of disease of the blood vessels to the brain) may lead to terrible disability. Damage to the blood vessels elsewhere in the body can make exercise difficult and limit mobility. There is no doubt that cardiovascular disease shatters lives, but there are many things that you can do to prevent cardiovascular disease, or reduce your risk of a heart attack or stroke.

Start by stopping smoking to keep your blood pressure under control and look at ways of reducing high cholesterol levels. It is also important to keep your size and shape healthy. An apple shape with a big tummy is particularly linked to cardiovascular disease. Measure your waist circumference rather than weight, and aim to keep it below 35 inches (89 cm) for women and 40 inches (102 cm) for men. You can help keep a healthy shape by exercising frequently. To protect your heart, you need only do 30 minutes of a moderate-intensity activity on most days of the week. But make sure you eat a healthy diet, otherwise all that exercise will go to waste. Another measure you can take is to ask your doctor about specific dietary supplements to boost the levels of essential micronutrients in your body—research has shown, for example, that the risk of heart disease is more than 30 percent lower among people with a high intake of folate or vitamin B6. Not surprisingly, stress

THERE ARE MANY THINGS THAT YOU CAN DO TO PREVENT CARDIOVASCULAR DISEASE, OR REDUCE YOUR RISKS.

can also have a bad effect on your heart, so learn to deal with it. If you suffer from diabetes it is important to manage this. And finally, ask your doctor about preventative medicines such as the polypill.

The polypill

In 2003, researchers at London's Wolfson Institute of Preventative Medicine proposed a "polypill" that contained six different drugs to lower the four key risk factors in cardiovascular disease. They said that the polypill should be given to everyone over the age of 55, and claimed that it could slash the rate of deaths from heart attack or stroke by more than 80 percent. Those people who started taking it at 55, they said, could expect to gain an extra 12 years of life. Testing of the polypill itself is ongoing and similar combination-drug treatments as an approach to prevention continue to be heavily debated.

17

FIND YOUR COMMUNITY

Human beings are inherently social creatures—our minds and bodies were designed to work best when we live together in a group and support each other through the normal stresses of life, whether simply gathering food or facing an enemy. Being isolated, on the other hand, especially after divorce or the death of a partner, is linked to an increased risk of loneliness, depression and personal neglect.

Supportive social relationships improve your well-being: People who are more involved in their community have a better social support network, which helps them stay healthier and live longer than those who live alone.

How to get involved

- Join a club and meet people who share your interests.
- Go regularly to the local gym or sports center.
- Volunteer—start doing things for others and everyone will want to be your friend!
- Use local shops and services, and get to know your area well.
- Spend some time walking or just enjoying the buzz around you in a nearby park or nature reserve.
- Choose a peaceful evening to sort out your finances, and if they look too chaotic to sort out yourself, get help from a financial advisor.

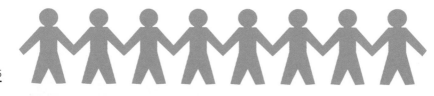

18

LAUGH A LOT

You might instinctively imagine that laughing a lot has to be good for you. Though research hasn't yet been able to conclusively prove this, laboratory experiments do suggest that being exposed to comedy may slightly improve your immunity to disease or reduce the amount of pain you feel. However, despite the fact that laughter is often used as a way to defuse stress, there is little evidence that it can actually improve physical health in the long run.

HAVING FUN MAKES YOU FEEL GOOD AND IMPROVES THE OVERALL QUALITY OF YOUR LIFE.

But don't be put off, because having fun definitely makes you feel good and improves the overall quality of your life. There is even humor therapy and clown therapy, laughter yoga, and laughter clubs for those who find it difficult to bring laughter into their lives spontaneously.

ENJOY CHOCOLATE

The occasional dark chocolate treat can do much to lift the spirits and may even have an aphrodisiac effect. The notorious Italian lover Casanova was in no doubt about the erotic effects of drinking chocolate, describing it as "the elixir of love". As well as prompting the body to make the "feel-good" hormone serotonin, chocolate also contains phenethylamine, a chemical that, if taken in large enough quantities, would have the same psychotropic effects as drugs such as opium and LSD. Phenethylamine is quickly metabolized in the body, preventing large concentrations from reaching the brain, but it leaves us with the sense of wellbeing that many of us have associated with chocolate since childhood.

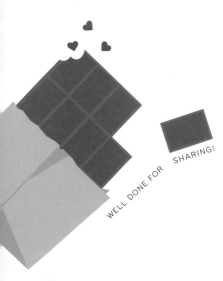

WELL DONE FOR SHARING!

CARRY ON LEARNING

Don't stop learning once you leave school. Keep stretching your mind, as learning forces the brain to grow new connections between the nerve cells—a direct antidote to aging. Pick up that electric guitar you have always wanted to play, learn tenpin bowling or how to become an expert at growing pumpkins. Even a simple change in routine—cooking a new recipe or taking a different route home from work, for instance—can help to keep your brain on its toes.

KEEP STRETCHING YOUR MIND. EVEN A SIMPLE CHANGE IN ROUTINE CAN HELP TO KEEP YOUR BRAIN ON ITS TOES.

In a study started in 1993 by Rush University Medical Center in Chicago, for example, those who said that they spent time on activities involving significant information processing (such as listening to the radio, reading newspapers, going to museums, doing crosswords, or solving puzzle games) had nearly half the risk of developing Alzheimer's disease as those who did not.

And if you keep your mind active as you get older, you are more likely to keep your body active, too, and avoid the onset of dementia and other related conditions.

21

MINIMIZE STRESS

Stress is the thread that pulls together a web of factors that affect your well-being.

When you feel stressed your brain senses danger: its "fight or flight" response urges into action various mechanisms in your body that release adrenaline, and raise your heart rate and blood pressure, as well as unleashing the stress hormone called cortisol. This process is helpful at the instant you need to confront a threat, but if stress persists in the long term, it can start to cause damage to the body.

Some research has shown that continual elevated cortisol levels seem to kill cells within the hippocampus, an area of the brain that controls memory. Cortisol also reduces the brain's ability to make new neurons or nerve cells, and can generally cause premature aging of the brain. In addition, it changes the fats in the blood, which, combined with elevated blood pressure, greatly increases the risk of a heart attack or stroke, and may also have a negative effect on the immune system. Dealing with the stress in your life will improve your health and longevity in a multitude of ways.

Easier said than done, the key to reducing stress is recognizing what causes it. Identify areas of your life that regularly cause you anxiety. Simply identifying the stresses is a positive step in itself. Equally, accepting that some degree of stress is a normal part of life is another step in the right direction.

THE KEY TO REDUCING STRESS IS RECOGNIZING WHAT CAUSES IT. SIMPLY IDENTIFYING THE STRESSES IS A POSITIVE STEP IN ITSELF.

In order to minimize stress you need to work out which stresses you think you could cut down. Start by looking at different areas of your life: home, work, your relationships, or your finances, for example, and think about what you can do to reduce the stressful situations that occur.

Some people use negative stress-management techniques such as denial, overeating, binge drinking, taking drugs and smoking. Avoid these as much as possible as they are short-term solutions. Instead, find positive stress-management techniques that suit you, such as taking time out for artistic expression, relaxation, massage techniques, exercise, or talking problems through with a friend or a counselor.

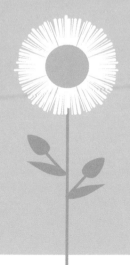

STRETCH YOURSELF

Limbs that are stiff are more prone to injury, and put abnormal strain on other areas of the body, leading to back pain, arthritis, and other problems. A lack of suppleness can cause tightness of the hamstring muscles in the leg, which is often a major factor in back pain and knee conditions.

Flexibility protects the muscles and joints from injury, reducing the risks of torn muscle fibers (strains) and torn ligaments (sprains). It helps to make exercise easier, allowing the musculoskeletal system to develop stamina and become strong. Being supple and lithe improves our sense of wellbeing; movement doesn't seem to be such a struggle, bending and stretching become effortless, and you want to get out there and dance (or run, jump, or play tennis—whatever you like).

Forward bend pose

Forward bends give an excellent stretch to the whole of the back of the body. They tone the abdominal organs and the kidneys, improving digestion and circulation.

- Start seated with your legs straight out in front of you and your feet hip-width apart and bend forward over your legs.
- You may find this pose difficult to begin with so try looping a strap around your feet to help you to hold it.
- If you can, hook your big toes with your index finger.
- Do not bounce in the pose and take extra care if you have back problems or sciatica.

TRY YOGA

According to yoga philosophy, it's the flexibility of the spine, not the number of years, that determines a person's age. Yoga slows down the ageing process by giving elasticity to the spine, firming up the skin, removing stress from the body, strengthening the abdominal muscles and correcting poor posture. The deep rhythmic breathing in yoga relieves respiratory complaints including asthma, while the increased oxygen boosts muscle strength.

Yoga is said to affect all the important determinants of a long life—the brain, spine, internal organs, and circulation—and to have a marked effect on pituitary, thyroid, adrenal, and sex glands. What is certainly true is that the relaxation techniques and physical exercise involved in yoga result in a positive mental and emotional state, making you feel more energized, relaxed, and generally optimistic.

The Sphinx

- Lie on your front, and place your elbows and hands on the floor with your back slightly arched.
- Relax into this position and press your hips into the floor. This stretches the front abdominal muscles and you may feel some movement in your lower back. If you have no pain in this position, you can move on to the next stage.
- Press on your hands, and lift your elbows off the floor, arching your body further back. Hold this position for 15 seconds, and then slowly release.

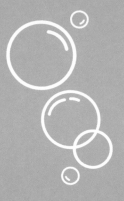

WASH YOUR HANDS

Only half of us wash our hands after visiting a public bathroom, and yet contact between people is the main way diseases spread. Even with diseases such as colds and flu, where we cough and sneeze viruses into the air, it is touching other people or their things or holding door handles that are contaminated by others, that is the main route of transmission. Wash your hands, and you wash away the risk of disease.

How to wash your hands

- Wash with soap and clean running water for at least 20 seconds— and don't skimp on the soap! (Alternatively, use an alcohol-based cleaner and rub until hands are dry.)
- Make a lather and scrub all surfaces of your hands, fingers, and wrists.
- Rinse hands well under running water.
- Dry your hands on a paper towel, then use it to turn off the tap. Or dry with a hand dryer.

When to wash your hands

- After using the bathroom.
- Before and after changing a baby's diaper or potty-training a child.
- Before preparing or eating food.
- After blowing your nose or sneezing.
- Before and after looking after someone who is ill.
- Before and after treating a wound.
- After handing animals or their waste.
- After handling garbage.
- After gardening.

GET SPORTY—SAFELY

Being active is an essential ingredient in any recipe for living longer. But if your choice of exercise is racing head-first down the Cresta Run on a skeleton toboggan then it could also be your downfall. While the thrill of an adventurous sport may offer that feel-good factor, a serious accident could also dramatically shorten your life. The Consumer Product Safety Commission in the US estimates that the highest numbers of sport-related injuries are from basketball (over 400,000 serious injuries a year), American football (the average age at death for an NFL pro is 55 years) and bicycling. In Australia, motorsports, horse riding, and power boating are the most dangerous, according to researchers at Monash University, Australia. And insurance companies levy the heaviest penalties on those who fly planes, climb mountains, hang glide, parachute, scuba dive, or take part in motorsports.

How to get active—safely
- Go slowly, and don't jump in at a level beyond your experience or capabilities. Work your way up to more adventurous activities.
- Always get expert advice and training.
- Wear the proper clothing, and use the proper equipment and safety gear.
- Follow the rules.
- Don't play if you are injured.

CREATE A MOLE MAP

Playing disease detective is quite straightforward when it comes to the skin. You'll particularly need to look out for the pigmented skin cancers called malignant melanomas as these can be very aggressive, spread quickly, and have a high mortality rate unless caught very early. Malignant melanoma has been increasing faster than any other type of tumor since the suntan became fashionable. To decrease your risk of developing skin cancer, protect yourself from UV light and keep an eye on your skin.

How to examine your skin

- It's important to check your own skin once a month. Self-examination is best done in a well-lit room in front of a full-length mirror.
- Check your face, ears, neck, chest, and stomach. Women will need to lift breasts to check the skin underneath.
- Check both sides of your arms, the tops and palms of your hands, and your fingernails.
- Sitting down, first check one leg, then the other. Inspect the bottoms of feet, calves, and the backs of thighs.
- Use a handheld mirror to inspect your neck, shoulders, upper arms, back, buttocks, and legs.
- Check for the following: A mole is more likely to be abnormal if a) one half of the mole does not match the other half; b) the edge of the mole is jagged or irregular; c) more than one color is present in the mole; d) it is larger than ¼ inch (5 mm) in diameter.

27

KNOW YOUR LIMITS

While a little might do us good, there's no doubt that alcohol in any great measure is a poison that can harm most of the systems of the body. And doctors are now learning how binge drinking—drinking large amounts of alcohol in a matter of hours or over a long weekend—may be particularly harmful, even when a person's overall alcohol intake is within recommended limits. And if it doesn't get your body, it may yet affect the rest of your life: Alcohol is a frequent factor in problems with family, relationships, work, finances, and crime. It's easy to see how drinking heavily can take years off your life.

How to drink more safely

- Stick to recommended limits: Most experts advise no more than three to four units of alcohol a day for men and no more than two to three units a day for women.
- Don't drink during pregnancy.
- Don't consume your entire week's allowance of units in one evening.
- Binge drinking, which produces very high levels of alcohol in the body, is far more toxic to the cells than if the same amount of alcohol were to be consumed at a slower, steadier rate, say over the course of a week.
- Never drink and drive.
- Try not to drink on an empty stomach: Food can help slow absorption of alcohol into the blood.
- Seek advice if you are worried about how much you drink.

KEEP THINGS CHEMICAL FREE

Our bodies are under a constant barrage of attack at a submicroscopic level by free radicals—these are essentially unstable atoms that react with nearby compounds in order to regain stability—which exist both in our bodies, and in the environment around us.

Within the body, free radicals are constantly being produced as a part of various metabolic processes. Some of these have a purpose: The cells of the immune system generate free radicals, for example, in order to neutralize invading viruses and bacteria. But free radicals can also cause damage to the cell's own components, such as the DNA or genetic material, or the proteins in the cell membranes. The resulting cellular damage is a central mechanism in the ageing process, as well as in diseases such as cancer, arthritis, cardiovascular disease, and Alzheimer's disease.

Environmental hazards—including radiation, and the chemicals in cigarette smoke, asbestos, coal, and herbicides—also increase our exposure to free radicals. Such environmental factors may provide an external source of free radicals, or increase free-radical production by the body itself. It has been calculated that the DNA in each cell suffers about 10,000 free-radical "hits" every day. The lungs are particularly vulnerable to free-radical attack because many chemical pollutants are inhaled. But free-radicals may also enter the body in the food we eat, or directly through the skin (as with radiation). Once in the body, the free radicals may trigger a sequence of activation of enzymes, inflammation, and release of chemical signals, which harms the tissues.

People who age well may have less oxidative free radical damage. On the Japanese island of Okinawa, where people seem to be particularly long-lived, research shows that people following traditional ways of life have lower blood levels of free radicals, possibly because of healthier lifestyles but also because of genetic variations that give them greater protection. To counteract the effect of free radicals, the body uses antioxidants—molecules that safely react with the free radicals to limit damage. But as we get older our antioxidant processes become less efficient, resulting in our need to actively take in extra antioxidant nutrients.

How to limit free-radical damage

Reduce environmental exposure:

- Avoid traffic exhaust fumes, which are high in cadmium.

- Steer clear of cigarette smoke (both first- and secondhand smoke).

- Reduce exposure to synthetic chemicals such as insecticides.

- Avoid heavy metals such as mercury, cadmium, and lead. Look out specifically for lead from old paint and pipes, high mercury levels in some fish (such as swordfish, tilefish, shark, and king mackerel), sewage sludge, fertilizers, pigments, and battery fluid.

- Avoid ionizing radiation from industrial pollution, sun exposure, cosmic rays and medical X-rays.

- Reduce production of free radicals in the body by avoiding high-fat, high-sugar, overprocessed foods.

- Increase intake of antioxidant nutrients.

BE AN EARLY BIRD

COCK A DOODLE DOO

From world leaders to influential scientists and artists, many successful people attribute their achievements partially to waking up early.

Adding just one extra hour to your waking day can have a positive impact on many aspects of your life:

- Waking up earlier gives you more time to exercise, energizing both your mind and body by increasing blood circulation.

- Arriving early at work and having a quiet, peaceful hour to focus will help you plan and prepare better for the day ahead, alleviating work-related stress, and increasing your productivity.

- Waking up earlier can also aid better sleep, as your body is tuned with the earth's circadian rhythms.

- Studies have shown that "morning people" are more optimistic, proactive, and better at solving problems efficiently.

WAKE UP!

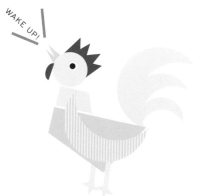

MAKE BOWEL-FRIENDLY CHOICES

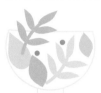

If you want to live forever, then you're going to have to abandon any inhibitions you might have about the business of your bowels. Making the top three on the list of common cancers, bowel cancer still proves fatal in about 50 percent of cases, despite modern treatments.

Think about the bowel-friendly changes that you may need to make to your lifestyle. Aim for a diet with less red and processed meat, and a lot more vegetables and fiber, as well as a higher fish and milk intake. Regular physical activity and weight control are also important for keeping the bowel healthy.

Be alert to signs of trouble, especially if you have a family history of bowel cancer. Ask your doctor about any applicable screening tests, like a genetic screening, colonoscopy or scans of the abdomen. Meanwhile, research shows that sending off a fecal sample for testing for occult blood (hidden bleeding) every two years can reduce your risk of dying from bowel cancer by 15 percent—a good return for a small, if rather unpleasant, task: about 50 percent of cancers detected this way are in the earliest stage, with a survival rate of greater than 80 percent. And if you develop symptoms such as a change in a regular bowel habit, or passing blood or mucus in the toilet, then get advice from your doctor urgently.

ACCEPT YOUR GENETIC DESTINY

The genes we inherit play a major part in determining how long we live. This is because not only do genes influence physical fitness, but also they shape our intellectual ability to understand what is necessary to stay healthy. Brain power, common sense, and personality—all strongly influenced by our genes—affect how we work to afford all those health necessities and fight off disease.

But the main genetic determinants of longevity are those that affect the way cells maintain and repair themselves. For example, centenarians have higher levels than the general population of a genetic product called PARP-1, a key chemical messenger involved in repair. People who reach 100 are also much less likely to carry genes associated with cancer, disease of the blood vessels, degenerative diseases of the nerves and brain, or diabetes.

However, genes ultimately account for only 25 percent of what determines longevity. Environment and chance can significantly overrule their powers, and most of us can do something to outmaneuver the influence of our genes.

How to make the most of your genetic destiny

- Study your family, and learn about the genetic influences you are likely to be carrying.
- Take lifestyle steps relevant to your genetics. If you carry genes that leave you with dangerously high cholesterol levels, you must make efforts from an early age to control your cholesterol intake and treat the high levels if necessary.
- Make sure you get regular screening for diseases to which you may be vulnerable.
- Follow good medical advice when you do develop disease.

GET A GOOD NIGHT'S SLEEP

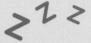

Good-quality sleep can be positively linked to successful aging and longer survival, while disruptive sleep patterns tend to be a sign of faster aging and disease. Sleep studies have shown that fragmented sleep raises levels of blood fats, cholesterol, cortisol, and blood pressure—all powerful risk factors for cardiovascular disease. Furthermore, lack of sleep reduces brain power and vigilance, leaving sleepy people prone to accidents during the day.

Some studies even suggest that sleep may be the most important predictor of how long you will live. A large study in the 1950s by the American Cancer Society found that the highest death rates were among those people who said that they slept for just four hours or fewer a night. Those who slept excessively—nine to ten or more hours a night—had higher death rates as well. More recent research has confirmed these findings, with those people sleeping six to seven hours a night living the longest.

How to get better sleep

- Stick to a regular sleep schedule, with the same bedtime every night, and a regular relaxing routine to help you wind down.
- Avoid late-night stimulants such as coffee, tea, hot chocolate and alcohol. Try herbal teas, especially chamomile, or milk instead.
- If you can't get to sleep after 20 minutes in bed, get up and sit quietly for a while before trying again. Don't watch TV or put on bright lights as this will tell your brain it's time to wake up.

HERBS FOR HEALTH

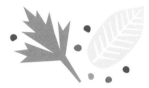

Cultivating herbs for culinary and aesthetic reasons is a popular activity, but it can also benefit your health, since herbs are packed full of nutrients.

Basil: Smelling a few basil leaves can help to relieve a tension or migraine headache and soothe menstrual symptoms. Consuming basil can ease bloating and stomach cramps.

Bay leaves: These contain laurenolide, an energizing ingredient, making them useful in a long-term detox program.

Coriander seed: This is used as an antibacterial treatment and to alleviate colic, neuralgia, and rheumatism.

Dandelion: This contains potassium, a diuretic, which extracts salt and water from the kidneys, so it is useful for anyone suffering from water retention.

Sage: Long considered a panacea for many health issues, sage is anti-inflammatory, antimicrobial, and is a good source of antioxidants.

Thyme: Thyme is loaded with antioxidants, including thymol, which has been shown to increase the number of healthy fats in cell structures. Thyme also helps to effectively relieve and treat nose and throat illnesses as well as digestive issues.

Mint: Cooling, calming and refreshing, mint eases stomach and digestive problems, relaxes the mind and relieves headaches.

Parsley: Packed full of vitamin C, parsley is a natural breath freshener. It also contains flavonoids, such as luteolin; these are powerful antioxidants that neutralize the free radicals produced by pollution, helping to prevent cell damage.

34

STAND TALL

Stop! Don't move—think about how your spine is shaped right now. Are you slumped over your desk? Uncomfortably perched on a chair? Is your pelvis crooked or twisted around your spine? If so, you could be putting your health at risk and chipping years off your life expectancy.

Now, sit upright. Plant your feet squarely on the floor and let your shoulders relax. Take some deep breaths. In these three short steps, you've taken positive action toward living a longer and healthier life. Doesn't that feel better? The body is a finely tuned piece of structural engineering. In order to work and move healthily, it needs to be fully aligned. A body out of line puts abnormal strain on the muscles, tendons, and ligaments, wearing out the joints, bones, and muscles and perhaps affecting the internal organs as well. Poor posture leads to lower back pain and arthritis, among other back and spinal injuries.

You can improve your posture at work by making sure your desk or work area is ergonomically designed. And get the advice of a physiotherapist, osteopath, chiropractor, or back specialist, who can advise you on exercises to align your bones and muscles. It's all about strengthening the muscles of your back and abdomen to hold your spine straight: Help yourself by asking a gym trainer for a special program, take up yoga, or try the Alexander technique.

Shoulder stretch:

- Stand a little away from a wall. Place your hands on the wall and walk your feet away until your upper body is horizontal, with back and arms straight and hands still pressing on the wall.
- Press your armpits toward the floor to feel a flexing in the shoulder joints. Press and release a few times to extend the range of movement of the shoulders.

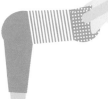

GET SOME SUN

We know enough these days about skin damage to slather on the sunblock and retreat from the sun, but in doing so, many people are now missing out on a vital ingredient for long life—vitamin D.

The body uses sunlight to make vitamin D; it uses, more specifically, the ultraviolet B (UVB) ray—the type of UV that causes burning and that is the major target for sunblock.

Meanwhile, vitamin D helps protect against a host of life-shortening conditions, including many common cancers, multiple sclerosis, rheumatoid arthritis, hypertension, cardiovascular heart disease, and Type 1 diabetes. Without sufficient vitamin D, the muscles become weak and the risk of falls and fractures spirals, especially in older people. For some people, lack of sunlight, especially in the winter, can lead to mood changes and depression, known as Seasonal Affective Disorder (SAD).

What is needed is a balance: Enough UVB to enjoy its health benefits, but not so much that it damages the skin. You will need to take into account season, latitude, time of day, and your skin pigmentation in order to work out what is right for you. But a rough guide to sensible exposure is 10 to 15 minutes of sun on the arms and legs, or the hands, arms, and face, two times a week, ideally avoiding the hours of maximum intensity of sunshine (that is, between 12 P.M. and 2 P.M.).

ALWAYS USE SPF

The main risk from sunbathing comes from the increase in skin cancers when people are exposed to intense UV light. The pigmented skin cancers called melanomas are the most sinister: They are aggressive, spread easily, and can be difficult to treat.

The photoaging effect of UV light—and UVA rays—is significant if you want to retain a youthful look. A suntan is really a sign of the burning of the epidermis (top layer of skin). With continued exposure to the sun, skin becomes thinner and more fragile, and its connective tissues weaken, reducing strength and elasticity. Skin damage shows up in deep wrinkles, fine veins across the cheeks and nose, and patches of pigmentation such as tiny freckles and "liver spots." These are hard to avoid, but you can limit or slow the damage by protecting your skin from excessive doses of UV light.

How to protect your skin from the sun

- Cover up with suitable clothing.
- Wear a broad-brimmed hat or stay in the shade.
- Apply high-protection sunblock liberally and frequently.
- Avoid the strongest sun in the middle of the day.
- Avoid such intense UV that you get sunburn, especially in childhood.
- Avoid sunbeds and lamps.
- Get all strange spots and moles checked out early.

EAT MAGIC MINERALS

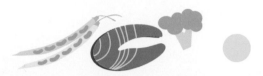

Besides playing various vital roles in the healthy functioning of your body, minerals keep the immune system working well. However, as we get older, we are more likely to become deficient in certain minerals because of poor diet, increasing needs, or excess loss from the body. Mineral deficiency may play a part in many life-shortening diseases. For example, people with a lower magnesium intake, are more likely to develop Type 2 (non-insulin-dependent) diabetes while low levels of selenium are linked to poor immune function and an increased risk of cancer.

Magic minerals include calcium for good bones, iron to transport oxygen in the blood, selenium to make certain enzymes, magnesium to help important biochemical reactions in the body, and zinc to slow age-related deterioration of cells.

How to increase your intake of minerals

- Start by eating a wide variety of foods, as different minerals are found in different foods. You could get calcium from dairy products and fish such as salmon and sardines; iron from red meat, eggs, beans, and leafy green vegetables; and zinc from meat and legumes.
- Buy organic: Modern farming and food preparation can deplete levels of certain minerals.
- Take a daily supplement if you or your doctor think you need it.

BRUSH YOUR TEETH

Good dental care could actually help you live longer by preventing other common killers, according to the American Academy of Periodontology. Our mouths are full of bacteria that may be harmful if they get into the bloodstream. Healthy gums help form a barrier that the bacteria cannot cross, but if we don't look after our gums an infection known as periodontal disease can set in, breaking down the defenses, and allowing the bacteria an easy route to enter the body. Recent research has linked periodontal infections to heart disease, diabetes, and respiratory disease. Unfortunately, too, the risk of periodontal disease increases as we get older, raising the general level of inflammation in the body.

Remember to take care of your teeth and gums by brushing frequently and thoroughly, flossing properly, and seeing your dentist regularly. He or she will also be able to spot if you develop cancer of the mouth or oral cavity.

LISTEN TO YOUR DOCTOR

Medicines can have a dramatic effect on keeping disease at bay, and prolonging both health and life expectancy. Your doctor will prescribe a drug based on a sound knowledge of what benefits it can bring. But many medicines, especially those for chronic problems such as diabetes or high blood pressure, usually need to be taken carefully, as prescribed, every day for the rest of your life. People often forget, or can't be bothered with their pills, or can't cope with the side effects but don't go back to their doctor to talk about the problem. As many as 25 percent of prescriptions for medicines are never taken to the pharmacy to be filled, and even when they are, many more are just left on the shelf at home, and never taken as recommended.

READ THE LABEL, NEVER DOUBLE DOSE, AND GET BACK TO YOUR DOCTOR IMMEDIATELY IF THINGS DON'T SEEM RIGHT.

A study of heart attack survivors in Toronto, Canada, showed a higher death rate for those patients who were particularly bad at taking their medicines after the attack. But you don't need a scientific study to tell you that your prescribed pills aren't doing you any good just sitting in their bottles!

However, research has also shown that the more medicines you need to take, the greater the chance that there will be a medical error of some sort. Older people taking three or four drugs a day are more than twice as likely to make a mistake; if you need seven medicines each day, the risk of errors is tripled. Always read the labels of your medicines and follow the instructions meticulously. Never double dose or take medicines prescribed for someone else. And get back to your doctor immediately if things don't seem right.

DO GOOD DEEDS

Doing good deeds for others not only boosts your mood at the time, but also leads to long-lasting happiness. Scientific studies show that acts of kindness have more of an impact on your well-being if you do a variety of different things rather than repeating the same activity on a number of occasions. Researchers have suggested reasons why performing acts of kindness for others increases happiness. These include feeling more confident, in control, and optimistic about your ability to make a difference; for instance, volunteering enables you to connect with other people, and may help you feel more positive about the community in which you live.

DOING GOOD DEEDS NOT ONLY BOOSTS YOUR MOOD AT THE TIME, BUT ALSO LEADS TO LONG-LASTING HAPPINESS.

FIND SOME QUIET TIME

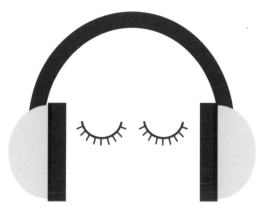

Turn down the sound, or tug on some ear muffs—noise pollution is a significant factor contributing to the premature death of people throughout the world, according to the World Health Organization (WHO).

One of the most important links is between noise and the developed world's number-one killer, heart disease. Long-term exposure to traffic noise has been blamed for as many as 3 percent of deaths from coronary heart disease, or more than 200,000 deaths each year around the world.

Meanwhile, low-level background noise all around the clock, which most people recognize as irritating and depressing, can also raise stress levels, and may be responsible for just as many early deaths as loud noise. A mere 35 decibels of background noise is enough to annoy and raise the risks. And night time noise may have an impact through its disruptive effects on sleep, so increasing fatigue, irritability, and aggression.

A GLASS A DAY

Some years ago researchers noticed that the French, despite eating lots of fatty foods, have low rates of cardiovascular disease. Although they drank five times as much red wine as their neighbors in the U.K., they were four times less likely to die from heart disease. Since then, several studies have shown that drinking one to two units of alcohol a day is linked with better health and longevity.

Research suggests that the polyphenolic compounds found in red wine interfere with the formation of atherosclerosis (fatty deposits that "harden" the arteries), helping to keep the blood vessels healthy. Many of these polyphenolic compounds have an antioxidant effect, which may explain why a moderate intake of alcohol could also be linked with a lower risk of cancer. Though the findings are still under discussion, a little tipple is unlikely to do you any harm, and could well help you live a longer life.

Know your units
- One unit of alcohol is 0.3 ounces (8 g) of alcohol and is typically described as:
  - One small glass of wine; or
  - Half a pint of any average-strength beer; or
  - A bar or pub measure of spirits, such as gin or whiskey

Note that drink strengths vary, as do pub measures and wine glass sizes, so these are just a rough guide.

TAKE YOUR OMEGA-3S

Truly nature's own wonder workers, omega-3s, an important group of polyunsaturated fatty acids (PUFAs), are essential for growth and development. They do a fantastic job of preventing coronary heart disease, high blood pressure, diabetes, and arthritis, among a host of other conditions.

Humans evolved on a diet that contained roughly equal amounts of omega-3 and omega-6 fatty acids. But this balance has gone out of kilter in the last couple of centuries: We now consume as much as 20 or 30 times more omega-6s than omega-3s, partly because of the increased amount of certain vegetable oils in our diet. This shifts the physiology of the body to a state where blood is thicker, blood vessels are more likely to go into spasm, and clots are more likely to form. Although omega-3s counteract this effect, reducing inflammation and thrombosis, we are generally not getting enough for them to do the job right.

How to increase your omega-3 intake:

- Oily fish such as mackerel, salmon, or sardines are a good source and you should aim to eat at least two portions a week.
- Replace sunflower, safflower, sesame, and corn oils with flaxseed, walnut, and canola oils, which are richer in omega-3 alpha-linolenic acid.

o-mega good

BALANCE YOUR HORMONES

Levels of many hormones in the body fall with age. As these hormone levels fall, and symptoms of disease appear, there is a clear justification for trying to replenish those failing hormones. But the scientific evidence to prove the benefits of hormone replacement therapy (HRT) is controversial. Since the 1990s, many wide-ranging studies have been carried out examining the effects of replacing female sex hormones for women going through menopause; the evidence remains inconclusive—in some cases even directly contradictory—on how effective HRT actually is, and the debate continues.

The evidence for most other types of HRT is also unclear. There have only been small studies of healthy older adults taking human growth hormone, for example, and these found that while injections may increase muscle mass and reduce body fat, they don't actually increase strength: Strength training is a cheaper and more effective way to achieve this. Neither is it clear whether human growth hormone can provide other benefits to healthy adults, such as increased bone density and improved mood. Side effects are also a problem, so beware the sales hype.

Levels of testosterone in women drop gradually with age, but the levels decline more substantially after a hysterectomy and oophorectomy. At this time, HRT is used in the form of one or more female hormones of estrogen and progesterone for menopausal symptoms, or severe hot flashes. Make sure to get expert advice relevant to your health problem first, before starting any hormone supplements.

How to be informed about your health

- Levels of many hormones in the body decrease with age.
- Levels of the female sex hormones estrogen and progesterone drop during menopause. The genital tissues thin, increasing the risk of urinary tract infection, while the risk of osteoporosis and heart disease increase.
- Quantities of growth hormone (GH) and testosterone are diminished, which may result in a decrease in lean body mass and an increase in adipose tissue.
- The pancreas becomes less efficient at producing the hormone insulin, which can lead to diabetes.
- Levels of dehydroepiandrosterone (DHEA), a hormone that is produced by the adrenal gland and is the main precursor of the sex hormones, fall steadily.
- Levels of thyroid hormones can wane, leading to problems such as tiredness, depression, constipation, and dryness of the skin and hair.
- Levels of melatonin may decline, disrupting control of normal body rhythms, and resulting in possibly a deterioration of immunity.

FIND YOUR HAPPY

Research has found that happy people act in healthier ways, getting more exercise, and taking part in more social activities than unhappy people do. Positive emotions appear to mean quicker recovery from illness by boosting the immune system, a longer life, and less chance of disability.

In one study conducted by Cohen, Doyle, Turner, Alper, and Skoner in 2003, the least happy third of the participants were 2.9 times more likely to develop a cold than the happiest. Cancer patients who experience more positive emotions each day have higher levels of "natural killer" cells (which can destroy cancer cells). So find your happy and live well!

How to get happy

- Make a list of the sources of unhappiness in your life, and look for ways to deal with these.
- Make a list of the real joys in your life, and aim for a daily dose of one or more of them.
- Adopt the art of mindfulness; take pleasure from the simple things in life.
- Set yourself realistic goals and expectations.
- Take time for yourself.

TAKE A SIESTA

People living in the tropics traditionally take a siesta or short nap after lunch. It's a logical way to escape the intense heat of the midday sun, which can put strain on the body, raising blood pressure and heart rate. But are daytime naps really good for you? It's a subject of great debate.

TAKING REGULAR MIDDAY NAPS MAY HELP TO REDUCE THE RISK OF HEART DISEASE.

A study from Greece showed that regular midday naps of about 30 minutes may help reduce the risk of heart disease, especially in men, possibly because they help to break the tension of the day, and relieve stress. In the study people who napped at least three times a week for almost 30 minutes had a 37 percent reduction in the risk of dying from a heart attack, or another heart-related problem.

However, a longer nap can disrupt your daily sleep pattern and alter the quality of sleep at night. It may also be a sign that night time sleep is inadequate, for example, because of potentially fatal conditions such as obstructive sleep apnea. If you find you need more substantial snoozes during the day, it may be time to get your health checked out.

BEAT STATUS SYNDROME

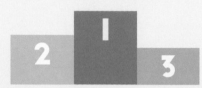

ADOPTING THE SELF-ASSURANCE OF YOUR SOCIAL SUPERIORS MAY HELP YOU TO LIVE A MORE SATISFIED LIFE.

Social status can be a prickly issue, but overwhelming evidence points to longer lives for people with a higher social standing, rank, or position. It's called "Status Syndrome" and, according to epidemiologist Sir Michael Marmot, the pattern is repeated across all groups in society, throughout the world, from the most disenfranchised to the leaders of our nations.

It's difficult to explain why status keeps us going. The links between social class—which contributes to status—and life expectancy are strong and becoming stronger. By the end of the twentieth century, professionals such as doctors and lawyers could expect to live, on average, nearly 1,500 days longer than unskilled manual workers. Key factors may include a feeling of having control over one's life, the ability to participate fully in society, and the connection between being rich and feeling rich. Whatever the mechanism, scientists have found that people with low social status are biologically older than their higher-ranking peers, as their genetic material (DNA) is shortened or becomes more frayed.

While you may not be able to think yourself rich, adopting the self-assurance of your social superiors may help you to live a more satisfied life, if not necessarily a longer one.

KEEP WALKING

Exercise can reduce the risk of heart disease, diabetes, colon cancer, and breast cancer, and generally keep death at bay. The Harvard Alumni Study, carried out over 38 years, concluded that a brisk, hour-long walk five days a week nearly halves the risk of having a stroke. Even walking for half an hour a day five times a week drops the risk by 24 percent. Other research shows that just 30 minutes of exercise a day cuts the risk of breast cancer by half for postmenopausal women. Exercise sparks brain cells into action too: Walking (or dancing or swimming—the choice is yours) for just 45 minutes three times a week helps reverse the natural decline of your IQ.

Think you're too late to start? The Harvard study showed that people over 75 who took up exercise and quit smoking could add, on average, almost two years to their lives. And before you yell "I haven't got the time!" remember that something is better than nothing. You can break up your exercise into small chunks—half a mile here, a third of a mile there—as what matters is the daily total. Among those Harvard alumni who had no major health risk factors, a weekend-warrior approach to exercise (that is, just one to two episodes a week, generating a total of 1,000 calories) was enough to postpone mortality.

As American health motivator Robert Sweetgall says, "Get off your ass and start moving around!"

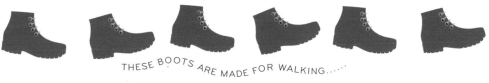

THESE BOOTS ARE MADE FOR WALKING......

49

ENJOY GOOD SEX

Shocking news! Sex is good for you! Research shows that the more often men experience orgasms, the lower their risk of dying. There's also evidence that men who ejaculate frequently are less likely to develop cancer of the prostate.

GOOD SEX MAY BENEFIT YOUR HEALTH. INTIMACY, COMFORT, AND PLEASURE ALL RELIEVE STRESS AND BRING HAPPINESS.

Some early research into sex and health has suggested that while frequency of sex is associated with mortality in men—the Swedes discovered, for example, that once men give up having sex they are more likely to die—it is the enjoyment of sex, rather, that is linked to death rates in women. Studies have found that women who don't enjoy a fulfilling sex life because their partners have problems with premature ejaculation or impotence, are more likely to have a heart attack.

The available research backs up the common belief that what matters a lot for men is how often they have sex—the physical activity may be most important—but for women, the quality of the emotional experience may have greater value. It is easy to imagine how good sex, especially within a stable relationship, may be good for your health: Intimacy, comfort, and pleasure all relieve stress and bring happiness, while the physical effort gives the cardiovascular system a good workout. So get it while you can!

50

KEEP IT SAFE

We've found that sex is good for you—so why ruin its positive effects by catching a sexually transmitted disease (STD)?

If you have unprotected sex, you will be at risk from sexually transmitted infections such as HIV. The risk is even greater if you have frequent, casual partners.

While ever-improving medical treatments mean that HIV isn't the death sentence it once was, it still can't be cured. Modern treatments can keep the virus under control, and limit the damage that it does, but they can have troublesome side effects, and the virus may become resistant.

HIV isn't the only STD that you need to protect yourself from. Other potentially fatal viral infections such as hepatitis B and hepatitis C may be passed on during sex, with serious implications for long term health. As many as 70 percent of people with hepatitis C, for example, will develop chronic liver disease, and up to 5 percent will die as a result.

How to avoid STDs
- Discuss STDs with your partner(s) and consider getting tested before having sex.
- Protect yourself with condoms and avoid sex while under the influence of drugs and alcohol, which can impair your judgement.
- Talk to your doctor about vaccinations for human papillomavirus (HPV) and hepatitis B.

BOOST YOUR VITAMIN INTAKE

The need for vitamins has been recognized for centuries—the ancient Egyptians knew that eating liver could prevent night blindness (now known to be due to vitamin A deficiency), and lemons and limes were first used by the British Royal Navy in the eighteenth century to prevent scurvy (a disease caused by vitamin C deficiency).

We know that minute amounts of vitamins are required in our diet for essential metabolic processes within the body, and that they are vital for health, as without them we are vulnerable to disease. But scientific research has as yet been unable to determine whether taking supplemental vitamins offers particular health benefits.

Governmental guidelines suggest the amount of each vitamin that you should get in your diet every day, and eating a good balance of foods should ensure that you get adequate amounts of the vitamins you need. But some people argue that these recommended allowances are simply a measure of what is enough to keep at bay those conditions recognized to be the result of vitamin deficiencies, rather than proposing an amount to actively promote health in other ways—by improving the immune system, for example. As many studies have conflicting findings, the evidence isn't yet clear that higher levels of many vitamins can definitively prolong the human life span. Stay on top of the most recent Recommended Dietary Allowance (RDA) recommendations and discuss taking additional supplements with your doctor.

HAVE A STAYCATION

Vacations are great opportunities to visit different cities or countries but more often than not we ignore the communities that we live in. Instead of paying hundreds or even thousands of dollars for an exotic trip, consider taking a "staycation". On your staycation, you can explore the parts of your community that you've never been to before. Try a new restaurant, visit local art galleries and museums, or have a picnic in the park—hopefully by the end you will be looking at your hometown with a refreshed perspective.

Staycations are also a wonderful chance to catch up on housework or errands. They allow you to relax and enjoy yourself in a familiar setting, without the added pressure of booking hotels, catching flights, or adapting to new time zones.

USE YOUR STAYCATION TO TRY A NEW RESTAURANT, VISIT LOCAL ART GALLERIES AND MUSEUMS, OR HAVE A PICNIC IN THE PARK.

BE RADIATION AWARE

The earth is naturally radioactive, as is the air you breathe, the food you eat and the ground you stand on. Modern technology adds to the radiation bank new risks from sources such as X-ray machines, nuclear power stations, and even everyday objects such as smoke detectors and photocopiers.

Ionizing radiation is used in radiotherapy treatment to kill cancer cells—so sometimes controlled radiation can help people to live longer. But usually it does harm, altering the way cells grow, function, or reproduce. Very large doses of radiation can cause tissues with a rapid cell turnover to die, resulting in often fatal skin burns, anemia, and loss of intestinal membranes. More relevant are the long-term effects from chronic exposure, the most important of which is an increased risk of cancer, especially lung and blood cancer (leukemia).

Natural sources account for 85 percent of ionizing radiation. These include the earth's crust, from which seeps radon, which is responsible for half of all radiation exposure. Also, rocks, soil, and building materials, from which emanate gamma rays. Food and drink are another source of radiation, because plants and animals take in radioactive materials with nutrients. Some foods such as Brazil nuts, tea, coffee, and bread are more radioactive than others.

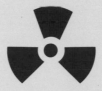

There are also important artificial sources of ionizing radiation, including medical tests and treatments, such as X-rays. On a larger scale, power stations, which release radioactive materials into the environment in gases (nuclear power) or ash (coal-fired power) are a source, as are nuclear power stations which discharge radioactive waste. But in reality, the risk of your exposure to radiation from power and nuclear stations is very small, even if you live right next to them.

How to protect yourself from ionizing radiation

- Avoid unnecessary exposure.
- Reduce exposure to radon.
- Don't have unnecessary X-rays.
- Limit the number of flights you take or trips to high altitudes.
- Be aware of any exposure through your job and take appropriate steps to fix this. Research has shown, for example, that pilots who have clocked more than 5,000 flying hours may be at increased risk of acute myeloid leukemia due to cosmic radiation at high altitudes.
- Know the risk from your local environment—be aware, for example, of any local industries releasing radioactivity into the rivers or air.

TRY MEDITATION

Meditation has been recommended for centuries as a natural path to health and longevity. The psychological benefits of meditation are now more widely recognized the world over, and are even used in some hospitals to reduce stress associated with chronic or terminal illness.

MEDITATION CAN LIFT MOOD, DISPEL ANXIETY, AND BE USED TO BANISH NEGATIVE THOUGHTS AND PESSIMISM.

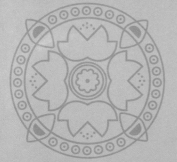

Studies of techniques such as transcendental meditation have shown that they can be effective in controlling blood pressure, keeping the arteries healthy and reducing the risk of heart disease. It can also be used for personal development and to focus the mind.

Those who meditate regularly say that it gives them an overall sense of peace and tranquility, which may be as restorative as sleep, and helps them escape from the pressures of a busy life.

Meditation can lift mood, dispel anxiety, and be used to banish negative thoughts and pessimism. People who meditate regularly also say that it helps them focus and concentrate, improving their performance at work, and bringing harmony to their relationships.

COLOR YOUR HOME

The colors you introduce to your home can have an impact on your well-being, since different colors are known to influence different emotions. And it is not just the colors that you use, but where you use them in the home, and how. When making your choice for a room, you may wish to consider the main emotional impact that specific colors are meant to have.

You can use just one main color throughout a room, or different tones of the same color. Alternatively, you can place extra splashes of "accent" color(s)—to complement a dominant color, or even equal amounts of two or more contrasting colors, making sure that there are no uneasy clashes. Objects that you should consider when matching or introducing a color scheme are soft furnishings (cushions, rugs, bedding); ornaments (framed photos, lamps, vases, sculptures); kitchenware (toaster, fruit bowls, tea towels); tableware (tablecloths, place mats, crockery); and floral arrangements, with endless color options.

Here are some common colors and their associations

- **Red:** Fiery and invigorating.
- **Orange:** Warm and reassuring.
- **Green:** Nourishing and soothing.
- **Blue:** Calming and cooling.
- **Yellow:** Sunny and uplifting.
- **Brown:** Grounding and practical.

56

BE SPONTANEOUS

Finding time to pursue your hobbies can be a challenge in your busy day-to-day life. However, by carrying some of your hobbies around with you, you can begin to experience them spontaneously. For instance, carry a book or knitting needles in your bag and make your rush-hour commute more enjoyable, or have a notebook and pen with you in case you observe something that you would like to write about or draw.

SPONTANEITY IS ABOUT KEEPING AN OPEN MIND TO LIFE'S POSSIBILITIES AND ACTIVELY EMBRACING NEW EXPERIENCES.

Spontaneity is also about practicing flexibility. If you make plans with a friend and they fall through, remember that it's not the end of the world. Think of ways to make the most of your freed-up time. And remember, spontaneity is not simply about diving off the steepest cliff; it is about keeping an open mind to life's possibilities and actively embracing new experiences.

BETTER TOGETHER

Both men and women live healthier, wealthier, happier, and longer lives when they are in a stable partnership. There is a huge amount of research showing a strong link between supportive social relationships and well-being.

In 2006, scientists from the University of California, Los Angeles, confirmed that married couples are more likely to live to an old age than their divorced, widowed, or unmarried counterparts. Their research showed that people who never marry are almost two-thirds more likely to die early, even though they appeared to be in better physical shape than their peers.

People who are happily married are less likely to have financial difficulties, or physical or mental health problems than those who aren't married. When illness does strike, being married may help speed recovery: Married people have been shown to have higher survival rates than single, widowed, or divorced people in some cancer cases, for example.

It appears there is something about marriage—a sense of belonging to a social institution, perhaps, or a public demonstration of shared aspirations—that gives it the edge over cohabitation.

WELCOME NEW CHALLENGES

Our lives today are driven by change—globalization, new technology, and the fast-moving nature of just about everything. People change too; our children grow up before our eyes and parents seem to age all too quickly.

Change in our lives is not just inevitable, it's an opportunity to grow and progress. Recognizing this as a fact of life can be liberating and life-changing. Rather than being daunting, all of this newness can bring excitement and interest into our lives. At the same time, it can help us master fresh skills, gain knowledge, and improve relationships.

Along with change come options, so recognize there will be unknowns and approach change positively with an open mind. Taking on new challenges, learning new skills, and developing interests in new directions can make a real difference to your happiness. Studies show that people who set goals that are designed to fulfill their potential as individuals, are likely to experience greater life satisfaction and less depression.

According to American psychologist Carol Ryff, people who score highly in personal initiative assessments exhibit the following characteristics:

- They are open to unfamiliar experiences and activities.
- They think it is important to have experiences that challenge the way they view themselves and the world.
- They are stimulated by the idea of continual intellectual growth.

CLEAN GREEN

We come into contact with thousands of different chemicals every day, in the food we eat and the cleaning products we use, in pesticides, packaging, toys, medicines and clothes, to name but a few items.

Although most cleaning products are labeled with known risks, other products in widespread use continue to cause problems ranging from allergies and asthma to infertility and a disruption of hormone levels. Seemingly innocuous activities may involve potentially hazardous chemicals: Fill up with gas, for example, and the fuel vapors at the pump will give you a dose of hundreds of potentially toxic hydrocarbons and additives, including benzene, which is known to be linked to leukemia. Or renovate your 1960s home and you may risk breathing in asbestos fibers from the building materials, which could cause a form of lung cancer.

In the quest for a long and healthy life, you should be aware of the chemicals in your environment and the risks they pose, as well as what you can do to reduce your exposure. Ecologically friendly or organic products may be the best way through our modern, chemically tinged world.

60

SEND A LETTER

Throughout history, great writers have revealed their lives, thoughts, and feelings through written missives. Letters can play a vital role in our modern lives, too. There's a special feeling of happiness and excitement we get when we open a personal letter. And sending a letter shows we care about the recipient, because it involves more time and effort than sending an email or a tweet.

You can also write letters to people in your life as a therapeutic practice. Instead of sending the letters, discard them after writing. This is a wonderful way to express your feelings without harming anyone else's

SENDING A LETTER SHOWS THAT YOU CARE ABOUT THE RECIPIENT BECAUSE IT INVOLVES MORE TIME AND EFFORT THAN AN EMAIL.

KEEP YOUR BRAIN ACTIVE

In order to stay well and live longer, we need to be able to look after ourselves, respond to sudden threats to our health, and understand and implement the long-term changes and actions that are needed to prevent or effectively fight disease. This requires brainpower. Sadly, dementia, a widespread problem throughout the world that becomes more common with advancing age, often slowly robs a person of their ability to care for themselves. Those afflicted with dementia withdraw from the world, eventually losing interest in eating, drinking, or moving, and become vulnerable to complications such as infection or falls. The disease also steals the enjoyment of life from many sufferers.

Dementia affects one in 20 people over 65, one in five over 80, and nearly one in two over 95. It can be viewed as a terminal disease because it is progressive, usually incurable, and limits life span, but you can take measures to reduce your risk. The higher the education level you achieve when young, the lower the risk of dementia later. And keeping your brain active as you get older—by learning new skills, for example—helps to prevent mental decline.

FIGHT DEMENTIA WITH FOOD

Make sure you are eating healthy foods. There is some suggestion that a diet full of antioxidants and oily fish at least once a week may help prevent dementia. A lot of research is being carried out into other dietary elements—curcumin, the main active ingredient of turmeric, may possibly help against Alzheimer's, for example, while ginkgo biloba might improve memory and overall function in people with dementia.

Some "superfoods" that may help keep your brain healthy

- Blueberries may protect the neurons in the brain from oxidative stress, and help prevent the decline seen in conditions such as Alzheimer's disease.
- Packed with omega-3 oils, salmon helps to improve memory, while reducing inflammation in the body and protecting us from various age-related conditions such as arthritis and heart disease.
- Broccoli contains a whole range of protective nutrients, including vitamin C, betacarotene, indole-3-carbinol (I3C), and sulphoraphane (which can protect against cancer), and also seems to protect the brain against decline.

EMBRACE THE
GRANDMOTHER EFFECT

On the one hand, the demands of having children may seem to suck every atom of your reserves, but they can also bring deep joy.

Evolutionary biologists call this the "Grandmother effect," whereby women have evolved to live until their children have successfully reproduced. Studies of large families in Utah have shown that women who have more children do not live as long as those with smaller families, and that those who have their children late in life, live longer. Research among the Sami women of Finland, meanwhile, has found no link to family size, but showed that women who had their last child at an older age lived longest.

Once they have helped their children through the difficulties of creating their own family (where, as the grandmother, they play an invaluable role in both teaching their child how to look after her newborn and in taking an active role in caring for their grandchild), their mortality rises steeply. So consider waiting a little longer to extend your family and reap the wellness rewards of being a grandparent at the same time as extending your own life.

MAINTAIN A GOOD
WORK–LIFE BALANCE

While some people thrive on a demanding schedule, and need a challenging occupation in their life, others find that a high-octane career leads only to burnout, stress, and depression. Everyone is different, and it is important to recognize this. Ultimately, the key is balance—and only you know where the balance lies.

Find the right job for you—have a career assessment if you think that will help. Whether you prefer to spend your time pruning plants in a nursery, or piloting a jumbo jet, you need to make sure your choice of work blends in with the other important areas of your life.

How to strike a good work–life balance

- Make a regular, honest appraisal of your job. Ask yourself if you look forward to work in the morning.
- If your work is starting to get you down, remember: It's never too late to stop and retrain in a new career.
- Don't forget that good communication is absolutely vital. Always be open with your family or partner about the ups and downs of your career to help balance your needs with theirs as well as to talk through your anxieties.

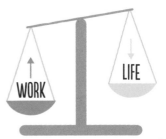

DRINK MORE WATER

Water accounts for almost two-thirds of our body weight, and is needed for every chemical reaction in our cells. It plays a vital role in metabolism, helping to absorb and transport nutrients, and to flush out waste products. Even minor dehydration can affect physical, mental, and emotional wellbeing. Our bodies lose water constantly through breathing, sweating, and passing urine, and we need to replace this to stay healthy. The total amount of water lost daily is about 3½ quarts (2.5 liters), but we get 1 quart (1 liter) of the fluid we need from food and the body recovers 10 fluid ounces (0.3 liters) through chemical processes. The rest must come from drinks. All nonalcoholic drinks count, but water, milk, and unsweetened fruit juices are the healthiest. To prevent dehydration, we should drink about 6 glasses (1.2 liters) of fluid every day.

USE ESSENTIAL OILS

Essential oils are a wonderful way to bring the healing benefits of aromatherapy into your life. They are versatile too: You can add them to a hot bath, use them to scent pot pourri, burn them in oil burners, or mix them in massage oils. Find essential oils at your local herbalist or pharmacy. Essential oils have surprising health benefits that can relieve everything from insomnia to skin problems.

Here is a short list of oils and their benefits

- Lavender: Known for curing insomnia and its ability to soothe frayed nerves. It can also be used to treat cuts and skin irritation.
- May Chang: Good for increasing energy, lifting mood, and beating depression.
- Calendula: Can be used to reduce the appearance of acne and scars, and is particularly good for sensitive skin.
- Oregano: Has potent antibacterial properties, which make it an effective fighter against colds and other sicknesses.
- Grapefruit: Great for boosting alertness and minimizing fatigue. Grapefruit oil can also be used in natural homemade cleaning products because of its antiseptic qualities.
- Eucalyptus: Good for fighting colds, relieving breathing problems, and stimulating the immune system. Only use it diluted, as undiluted it can irritate your skin.

ATTEND REGULAR SCREENING

The principle is simple: The earlier you catch a disease, the less damage it is likely to have done, and the easier it should be to treat. As a result it should have less impact on health expectancy, or longevity. Yet we often dismiss symptoms, delay getting expert advice, or hope the problem will go away. It's important to be vigilant for suspicious symptoms such as odd lumps and bumps, strange pains, rashes, the appearance of blood where it shouldn't be, or other changes in your body. Get advice from your doctor sooner rather than later about anything that is worrying you.

That said, many conditions march along deep inside the body without giving any clues to their existence. Undetected, a tumor may spread to the liver where it is more resistant to treatment, or the high pressure of blood may rip through the vessels to cause a devastating stroke. The only way to pick up the first stages of a number of conditions is to regularly screen ostensibly healthy people for early signs of them.

It is worth pointing out that screening can cause a lot of unnecessary worry about disease, especially when the tests used are not very sensitive, or produce false positive results which must be followed up with more invasive, potentially harmful tests that often show that there was nothing to worry about in the first place. So listen closely to the recommendations of your doctor—he or she can advise you on details such as how effective the test is, when it should be done, and how often it should be repeated.

Important screening tests

- **Breast cancer:** Genetic testing, mammogram, physical examination.
- **Prostate cancer:** Prostate specific antigen (PSA) blood test, rectal examination.
- **Cervical cancer:** Pap smear, DNA testing for high-risk types of human papilloma virus (HPV).
- **Bowel cancer:** Fecal occult blood (FOBT) test, flexible sigmoidoscopy.
- **Ovarian cancer:** Genetic testing, pelvic examination, ultrasound scan, CA-125 blood test.
- **Blood pressure:** Regular blood pressure measurements.

- **Heart disease:** ECG, exercise stress test, CT scan.
- **Diabetes:** Fasting blood sugar levels.
- **Thyroid disease:** Thyroid hormone levels in blood.
- **Kidney disease:** Kidney function blood test and urine analysis.
- **Stomach and duodenal ulcers:** Helicobacter infection test in breath, blood, or feces.
- **Glaucoma and other visual problems:** Dilated eye exam and pressure test.

. . . .

BE VIGILANT FOR SUSPICIOUS SYMPTOMS AND GET ADVICE FROM YOUR DOCTOR ABOUT ANYTHING THAT IS WORRYING YOU.

. . . .

68

BE A TEAM PLAYER

It's never too late to discover your inner athlete, even if you'll never play like a pro. Joining a sports team is a fun way to break out of your mundane exercise routine, and enjoy some social bonding. Many team players find that they enjoy it so much, it doesn't even feel like exercise. Team sports develop skills that are transferable to other parts of your life, such as decision-making, communication, and cooperation. Tennis, volleyball, bowling...pick one that appeals, and start building new relationships and social confidence at the same time as strengthening existing skills and building fitness. You're committed to a regular schedule of exercise, and to your team, so you're unlikely to lose motivation and give up. An added bonus—you'll bond with like-minded people and always have something to talk about.

Here are some of the best team sports to keep you fit

- Basketball: Varied movements use every muscle group in the body and fast running boosts the cardiovascular system.
- Rowing: A total body workout that sculpts and strengthens muscles in your arms, legs, back, and core.
- Soccer: Builds stamina, coordination, flexibility, and endurance through constant motion.
- Sailing: Improves nonverbal communication skills, while pulling and hoisting sails builds muscular strength and endurance.

GOOD VIBRATIONS

In 1993, the idea that listening to Mozart could boost your intelligence gained a great deal of attention after researchers found that 36 university undergraduates improved their ability to mentally manipulate objects in three-dimensional space after listening to 10 minutes of a sonata written by the great composer. Suddenly, the "Mozart Effect" was born, spawning a veritable industry of recordings that promised to boost intelligence. In the years since that first report the conclusions of the original research have often been overstated.

And yet, there are many researchers who still believe that listening to music can enhance your overall cognitive arousal, and your ability to concentrate. One Belgian group, for example, found that a music-based exercise program could improve cognitive function in a group of women with dementia.

In 2006, researchers reported in the Annals of the New York Academy of Sciences that listening to any music you find enjoyable has positive effects on cognition. So if you happen to enjoy Mozart, by all means play his music. If you don't, perhaps sticking to what you like might be more effective.

CATCH THE BUS

Switch from driving to public transportation for just one day and you'll make an immediate difference. A single person can save about 20 pounds (9 kg) of carbon dioxide per day, according to a study carried out by the American Public Transport Association. That adds up to about 2¼ short tons (about 2 metric tons) per year. A full underground train can remove more than 2,000 vehicles from the road. Because of its efficiency, many governments are actively pursuing public transportation as the only way to lower pollution, traffic, and greenhouse gases.

Here are some of the benefits of public transportation

- Public transportation reduces pollution.
- Using it produces 95 percent less carbon monoxide, about 50 percent less carbon dioxide and 50 percent fewer nitrogen oxides per mile compared to cars.
- Public transportation increases property values. Homes that are located near public transportation, and so linked to local amenities are often worth considerably more (studies show house prices increase by 13 to 45 percent depending on the city and neighborhood).
- Public transportation is also safer, according to the United States National Safety Council. Each mile travelled by car yields 25 times more fatal accidents compared to the same distance travelled on public transport. Injury rates are also lower per mile.

CUT DOWN ON FAST FOOD

Manufacturers face considerable challenges to prepare foods that will taste good, have a reasonable shelf life, and return a good profit. To manage this, they pack foods with preservatives, refined sugar, and hydrogenated or trans fats—ingredients that would make a nutritionist shriek.

And for good reason: In experiments, monkeys fed a fast-food diet rich in trans fats grew fatter around the waist than those fed a diet containing the same number of calories overall while being rich in unsaturated fats. The monkeys on the fast-food diet also developed signs of insulin resistance, an early indicator of diabetes. After six years, the trans-fat monkeys were 7.2 percent heavier than before (compared to a 1.2 percent weight gain in the other group), and had 30 percent more fat in their abdomen, which is particularly linked to heart disease.

If you regularly eat fast foods or prepackaged foods, consider healthier nutritional options and substitute saturated fats for unsaturated fats, like nuts and fish.

IF YOU EAT FAST FOODS OR PREPACKAGED FOODS, CONSIDER HEALTHIER OPTIONS.

EAT LOCAL

There are some eating experiences you never forget. Sometimes it is those that are extremely painful: A Jalapeño bitten whole before realizing that it wasn't a bell pepper, or a spoonful of wasabi mistaken for guacamole. And then there are those food memories that stand out because the first bite sends a shiver of sensuous pleasure along your tongue and tastebuds, a frequent experience for consumers of local food.

For those uninitiated to buying produce locally, now is the time to make your way down to the nearest farmer's market and try the squash or tomatoes—whatever is in season. Then compare it to the lesser equivalents that have traveled thousands of miles from overseas to reach your grocery store. The difference in taste should be fairly obvious: A snow pea grown by a local farmer and never refrigerated will retain more of its delicate flavor than one shipped in a plane from Guatemala. You don't have to take my word for it—just ask any number of the world's top chefs who buy local food in order to have the best possible ingredients.

By eating locally you're not just getting food of a higher quality, you're also supporting your local farmers and producers. At the same time the fuel costs and emissions of transportation are virtually cut out, which can add up to a total carbon saving of 5000 lb (2275 kg) a year, just by having local food once a week.

If you live in a northern climate, eating locally is much harder in the winter than in the summer. There are also some foods, like tea and coffee, that probably don't grow anywhere near where you live. Some environmentalists cut out these foods anyway—the 100-mile (160-km) and 250-mile (400-km) diets specify the acceptable distance produce can travel for it to be deemed edible (the distances are based on the number of miles a farmer can travel on horseback in one day). But these diets are only for really hardcore converts. The purpose is to help the planet, not to make life unbearably difficult. Try eating locally grown food just once a week. By becoming part of the local-food market, you help the farmers who are trying to bring the freshest ingredients to our tables, most of whom go out of their way to make sure their food is produced in a sustainable way. And while doing your part for the planet, you get to please your palate too.

Statistics for imported food

- On average, fresh produce travels around 1500 miles (2415 km) from its source to your plate.
- A typical meal in the US contains ingredients from at least five countries outside the US.
- In the UK, half of the vegetables and 95 percent of the fruit are imported.
- In the US, 12 percent of vegetables and 39 percent of fruits are imported.
- 30 percent of the vehicles on our roads are currently transporting food.

THINK LIKE AN OPTIMIST

A well-known study by the Mayo Clinic in the early 1950s showed that optimists live about 8 years longer on average than pessimists.

Optimistic older people have better immune function than pessimists, so being hopeful may keep disease at bay. Optimism also helps you to deal with illness, while pessimists tend to believe that "nothing I do will matter" and are more passive about their health. Research has shown that optimism is very helpful in heart disease, for example, reducing the likelihood of angina and heart attacks. Similarly, hope is a powerful weapon for cancer patients, and can significantly increase how long someone survives.

How to become an optimist

- Learn to recognize and abandon negative forms of thinking.
- Avoid filtering (focusing only on negative things) and personalizing (blaming yourself for bad things).
- Avoid catastrophizing (always expecting the worst) and polarizing (seeing things as always good or bad, not shades of either).
- Look for the good things, no matter how small, and cherish them.
- Try to play down the bad things—deal with them and move on.
- Keep company with other optimists!

DECLUTTER

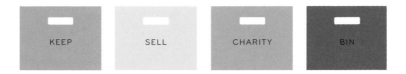

KEEP SELL CHARITY BIN

Creative clutter is one thing, but most people feel oppressed, stressed and depressed when they are surrounded by chaos. The stress of clutter is a powerful subliminal force that surreptitiously drives your autonomic nervous system, whether the mess is a jumble of material possessions, a muddle of outstanding debts or the turmoil of a tumultuous relationship.

Clutter can cause the pulse rate and blood pressure to simmer higher than is healthy, while adrenaline and cortisol do their damage. Figure out what kind of clutter you need to tackle, then get to work!

How to de-clutter
Clutter doesn't appear overnight, and won't go away quickly either. Set aside time to sort out every aspect of your life. If it's a messy space you're faced with, for example:

- Break down the mess into small chunks: Tackle a room, a cupboard or even a drawer at a time.
- Reorganize your storage space so that you can put things away and then easily find them again.
- Get rid of stuff you haven't touched in years—bring it to a thrift shop, give it to a friend, or have a garage sale.
- Get help: Ask a friend to help you sort the junk from the jewels!
- Choose a peaceful evening to sort out your finances, and if they look too chaotic to sort out yourself, get help from a financial advisor.

CONTROL YOUR WEIGHT

Countless studies have proven the link between weight and mortality, as well as poor quality of life. More acute levels of obesity introduce greater risks of suffering a heart attack or stroke, developing cancer or diabetes, or being afflicted with joint disease. Metabolic syndrome victims—obesity with high blood pressure, diabetes or insulin resistance, and abnormal cholesterol levels—are three times more likely to die earlier than normal for their age.

A 2006 National Institutes of Health study in the US compiled data from more than half a million Americans and found that even small increases in body mass index (BMI) can lead to premature death. In middle-aged men and women who had never smoked, simply being overweight (BMI of 25–30) was associated with a 20 to 40 percent increased risk for death.

The key to weight control is healthy eating and regular exercise—it's that simple. You should take steps such as measuring your weight once a week so you can't kid yourself. Find a sensible eating plan you can stick to—and avoid crash diets. Find exercise you enjoy and will keep doing. Make the most of available support, such as slimming groups and counseling. If necessary, you can also talk to your doctor about medical treatments for weight loss.

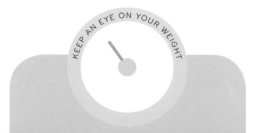

KEEP AN EYE ON YOUR WEIGHT

CHECK YOUR BMI

Being too thin isn't healthy either: Studies show that the risk of death rises as BMI drops below 24.5. In fact, studies carried out at the Institute of Preventative Medicine in Copenhagen found that women with wide hips were 87 percent less likely to die from heart disease than slim-hipped women. Fat in that area contains a natural anti-inflammatory chemical called adiponectin, which keeps arteries healthy; women with hips less than 40 inches (100 cm) wide don't get this protection.

How to measure your body mass index

The body mass index (BMI) measure

Divide your weight in pounds by your height in inches squared, and multiply the figure by 703. (To calculate your BMI in metric measurements, find your height in meters and square the figure. Divide your weight in kilograms by your height squared.) A normal BMI is between 18.5 and 25. A BMI above 30 indicates that you are obese and is associated with a greater risk of death. Note, though, that BMI doesn't distinguish between the weight of fat and that of muscle, so fit, muscular athletes may be misclassified.

Your waist circumference

Waist circumference is now thought to be a better indicator of body fat and risk than BMI. A circumference of more than 35 inches for women and 40 inches for men increases the risk of cardiovascular diseases and diabetes.

GIVE BLOOD

Blood donors are always in demand. It can take 50 units of blood just to save one car accident victim and five units of blood for one cancer treatment. Besides the obvious altruistic reasons for donating blood, studies have shown that it may also have health benefits for the donor. By having blood removed from your body, you also remove excess iron. Iron oxidizes cholesterol, which canlead to damaged arteries and heart disease. So roll up your sleeves for your heart, and somebody else's.

It's also beneficial to know your blood type as that will help you become aware of the health risks to which certain blood types may be predisposed. Also, if you're trying to conceive, knowing your own and your partner's blood type may help to avoid complications during pregnancy.

TRY A SUGAR DETOX

LOW SUGAR INTAKE CAN HELP CONTROL WEIGHT AND REDUCE RISKS ASSOCIATED WITH OBESITY.

Low sugar intake can help to control weight and reduce the risks associated with obesity. Furthermore, eating less sugar—and keeping a wary eye out for refined sugar in particular— may be an important part of the dietary-restriction strategy for improving health and prolonging life.

Cakes, cookies and fizzy drinks are full of sucrose, and even some "savory" processed foods contain more sugar than ice cream. Eating a high-sugar diet can cause tooth decay and excessive weight gain, which can lead to heart disease and type-2 diabetes. The British Dietetic Association recommends that "added sugars", including those in soft drinks and processed food, should not exceed 10 percent of total daily calorie intake. For someone consuming 2,000 calories a day, that would amount to 1³/4 ounces (50 g)—the amount of sugar in 2 cups (a half-liter bottle) of cola. So it's good to keep a close eye on the amount of sweet and processed food and drink that you consume.

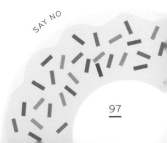

SAY NO

TAKE A BOX LUNCH

Making your own lunch and taking it to work has so many benefits. Firstly, it's usually healthier than buying a ready-made lunch. Secondly, it's far cheaper and can save you a lot of money over the year. And thirdly, it is better for the environment because it reduces packaging waste, which contributes to landfills and pollutes our oceans and waterways.

Make a commitment to set aside some time at the weekend, and prepare healthy food for lunches that you can freeze and pull out later. You can save more and eat more healthily by swapping meat for vegetables and pulses, which are nourishing sources of fiber, vitamins and minerals.

Leftovers from dinner are perfectly acceptable for lunch the next day, and they don't require any planning. Just make an extra portion or two of your evening meal, and put it in a portable container for reheating at work.

Here are some suggestions for nourishing and delicious packed lunches in winter

- Homemade soup with crackers or bread.
- Wholegrain pita bread with roasted vegetables and hummus (take a separate container and assemble at work).
- Hearty winter casseroles, stews, or curries.
- Small items to snack on through the day—fruit, nuts, hard-boiled eggs, carrot sticks, dried apricots, wholegrain crackers, low-fat yogurt.

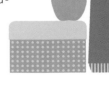

KNOWLEDGE IS POWER

When it comes to looking after your body and doing what you need to do to prevent premature aging, information is, undoubtedly, power. Ignorance is a fast track to illness and an early death. But an understanding of the particular health issues you face as you grow older will help to keep your engine running smoothly and allow you to spot the first signs of trouble. You also need to know how to separate the truth from the hype and to learn what doesn't work so that you don't waste your hard-earned cash on worthless anti-aging pills and potions.

Do you know what your cholesterol level should be and what it actually is? When was the last time you thought about your blood pressure? And do you know what screening you should be going for and how often? Just a few of the many questions that you need answers to if you want to live well. You're reading this book, so you're already on the right path!

How to be informed about your health
- Take power into your own hands and ask yourself these basic questions:
  - What are your cholesterol and blood pressure levels? What should they be? If they are high, what are you doing to bring them down?
  - Based on your age and family health history, what health screenings should you regularly schedule?
  - What health risks do you personally face—from your genes, your job, or your habits?

JUST SAY NO

There is a real risk of danger even with so-called "recreational drugs" such as cannabis, which some argue is not very harmful. While cannabis doesn't directly cause deaths, scientists are slowly discoveing the damage it can do. Cannabis smoke contains higher levels of cancer-causing substances than tobacco, and is inhaled for longer periods of time, for example. Research has shown that the highest risk of precancerous abnormalities in the lung occurs when cannabis and tobacco are smoked together. Significant and long-lasting psychotic effects can also occur. But, perhaps most importantly, the drug often introduces a person to the culture of substance abuse, which leads down a slippery slope to more harmful drugs and greater risks.

The dangers of drugs such as cocaine and heroin are more widely appreciated, as well as the links with other harmful behavior such as crime (in order to pay for a drug habit) or transmission of infections such as HIV and hepatitis C through contaminated needles. Steer clear of recreational drugs if you want to maximize your health—the consequences can be devastating.

NO TO DRUGS - YES TO LIFE

GET YOUR FIVE-A-DAY

According to the food pyramid that has been in existence in one form or another since the 1970s, your diet should include at least five portions of fruit and vegetables a day. This is to be balanced with six to ten portions of pasta, grains, and cereals; two to three portions each of protein and dairy foods and sparing quantities of fats and sugars.

In order to count toward your five a day, fruit and vegetables can be raw or cooked, frozen, canned or juiced. This may not seem such a tall order, but you might fail to achieve the quota day after day.

You should try to, though, because the health benefits of fruit and vegetables are substantial. Many of them are high in fiber and low in fat; they are packed with minerals, vitamins, and antioxidants. They have no artificial or added coloring or sweeteners.

In order to achieve your five a day, you should count on eating around 14 ounces (400 g) of fruit and vegetables a day. A medium-sized fruit (apple, banana) or two small fruits (kiwi, tomato) count as one portion, while two small vegetables (new potatoes, cauliflower florets) or three heaping tablespoons of cooked vegetables (corn, peas, beans) count as one portion.

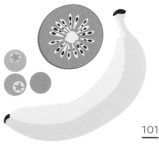

CATCH IT EARLY

Perhaps the main reason that a diagnosis of cancer is so feared, is that it almost inevitably brings a threat of death. But the impact of cancer on your life or health expectancy is hugely variable—you could lose a year or more of life expectancy for any sort of cancer other than non-pigmented skin cancer—and depends on factors such as the type of cancer, the location of the tumor, your age and general fitness, the treatment given, the expertise of the health professionals providing treatment, the occurrence of complications and other coincidental events.

Cancer of the pancreas, for example, is very aggressive and difficult to treat—only about 10 to 15 percent survive longer than a year after diagnosis, and only 2 to 3 percent are alive after five years. In comparison, survival rates in non-pigmented skin cancers are very high, and as many as 90 percent of people are cured and go on to enjoy a normal life expectancy.

Overall, it is estimated that about one in three people will be diagnosed with some form of cancer at some stage in their life. But cancer is predominantly a disease of ageing—below the age of 50 only about one in 27 people develop cancer. It becomes more likely as genetic damage accumulates over time, destroying the normal controls on cell division and growth. And as humans gradually live longer, so the proportion of people who develop cancer will increase. Information is power if you are diagnosed with cancer: Find out about different treatments and talk to your doctor.

HOW TO REDUCE THE RISKS OF CANCER

Avoid the known triggers.
- Give up smoking cigarettes or a pipe, or chewing tobacco.
- Avoid pollution and free radicals.
- Avoid excess sun exposure.
- Get more fruit and vegetables in your diet.
- Get enough nutrients in the form of vitamins, minerals, and antioxidants.
- Get plenty of fiber in your diet.

Exercise regularly.

Keep clear of radiation.

Take preventative medicines.

Aspirin has been shown to significantly reduce the rate of new polyps in people both with and without a history of colon polyps. However, taking aspirin to lower cancer risk should not been regarded as a substitute for established prevention tactics such as fecal occult blood testing and colonoscopy.

Get vaccinated against human papilloma virus.

This sexually transmitted infection is strongly linked to cancer of the cervix, vulva, anus, penis, and other sites.

Try to recognize symptoms of cancer early.
- Check your body regularly.
- Get expert advice concerning symptoms.
- Go for screening.

KEEP EVERYTHING
IN MODERATION

**WHAT WE EAT
AND DRINK PLAY
A VITAL PART
IN KEEPING US
HEALTHY.**

There is no doubt that what we eat and drink play a vital part in keeping us healthy. Experiments in dietary restriction since the 1930s have shown that restricting calorie intake extends life in a wide variety of creatures, including rats and nearly every invertebrate studied, such as worms and flies. But what about humans?

The facts are these: During normal aging, a progressive state of inflammation builds in the body, especially in the nervous system and brain. Dietary restriction is known to reduce the amount of inflammation in the body, and seems to increase the brain's ability to repair itself. If the theory of dietary restriction holds, eating less often, and/or fasting temporarily may eventually point to an extension of life.

You could try cutting down on calories or eating less frequently, but don't go overboard: A drastic reduction in calories and nutrients could damage the body, leaving your immune system shaky and vulnerable to infections and many other conditions.

Don't try sniffing at food to calm your appetite! Not only will it make you feel hungrier, but research on Drosophila fruit flies (which, strangely, age like humans) shows that simply the smell of food can significantly reverse the life-prolonging effects of calorie restriction.

FIND A GOOD CARE SYSTEM

If you want to age well, you're going to need your own personal health expert. A good doctor should understand your particular medical history and social issues, and should be able to recommend vaccinations or routine screening programs that may help to prevent cancer of the breast, colon, or cervix.

You need to have a good working relationship with your doctor so that you are comfortable asking about anything you need to know, without feeling embarrassed or as if you are wasting his or her time. If you don't like your doctor or don't get along well with him/her, it may be time to think about seeing someone else. Your doctor won't mind—we all understand that people relate in many different ways and we can't all get on with everybody else.

One of the best ways to find a good doctor is to ask your friends for a recommendation. It is also a good idea to check the doctor's qualifications and special interests, such as women's health or cardiology, to see if they match your likely needs or current conditions.

Once you have registered with a practice, when you meet your doctor, be honest with him or her—this is not the time to be shy or coy about health issues that may trouble you, however trivial you might think they are. It is also important that if you don't get on, you get out—and find someone else.

FIND YOUR BALANCE

In China and other Eastern countries you often see elderly people out early in the morning gently practicing tai chi in the local park. They are doing their best to avoid an event responsible for more deaths in older people in the western world than anything else—a fall.

Human beings are inherently unstable creatures. Walking on two legs we have a narrow base and a high center of gravity. To move without tumbling over, we normally rely on complex mechanisms that detect our state of balance and rapidly correct wobbles. While young we can lean, stumble, or trip and still finish upright. If we do fall, the worst result may be a fractured wrist, and this is a break that doesn't make much difference to life span. As we get older those mechanisms are increasingly likely to fail, and the chance increases of our ending up flat on the floor, even after the slightest challenge to our balance. Once you're over 65, you have a one in three chance of falling each year. With a loss of the necessary protective mechanisms, a fall can often result in a broken hip or a fractured skull. As the person is often left lying alone and with help beyond reach for hours, problems such as pneumonia, hypothermia, or dehydration may set in.

To reduce your chances of an early death by falling, you should follow a simple program of muscle strengthening and balance retraining. Take a tip from the east—refining your balance through exercises like tai chi can halve the risk of a fall.

QUIT SMOKING

Cigarette smoking is the single most important cause of preventable disease and premature death in developed countries. Tobacco smoke contains over 4,000 chemicals, many of which are highly toxic, such as arsenic, formaldehyde, cyanide, benzene, toluene, and acrolein.

Once smokers quit, their health risks rapidly drop, and within a few years they may almost be back to normal. For example, the risk of a heart attack for a quitter drops to the same level as a nonsmoker's within three years. And giving up cigarettes usually leads to considerable savings, reducing financial worries and allowing ex-smokers to enjoy more healthy pleasures, such as vacations.

How to quit smoking and stay a nonsmoker

- Believe you will be successful.
- Quit when you are in the right frame of mind. If you know you're having a bad week, it's not the right time.
- Don't go it alone—have a friend do it with you or join a smoking cessation program.
- Follow a structured plan—a smoking cessation clinic or program will help you create this.
- Make sure you have the necessary psychological support.
- Use medical treatments such nicotine-replacement therapy or anti-craving drugs as directed by your health professionals.
- Don't be discouraged if attempts to quit have failed in the past.

CONSUME GOOD FATS

Fat is an important part of our diet but if you want to avoid the Number 1 killer in the Western world—heart disease—you need to choose fats carefully.

When you think about fat in your diet, the aim should be to control the overall amount you consume (it's recommended that no more than 11 percent of calories each day should come from fats) and, more specifically, keep down levels of LDL-cholesterol, which is one of the worst criminals in cardiovascular disease. Saturated fat, trans-fatty acids (TFAs), and cholesterol in the diet all increase the risk of cardiovascular disease. TFAs may also raise levels of LDL-cholesterol ("bad" cholesterol) and reduce levels of HDL-cholesterol ("good" cholesterol). But mono- and polyunsaturated fats don't seem to have this harmful profile and may even help lower LDL-cholesterol slightly. How far eating the right fats will help you live longer is still being tested, but there is some evidence that it reduces heart problems and early death, so there is no harm in changing your habits for the better.

The main types of fat in food include saturated fat, which is found mostly in foods from animals and some plants, for instance butter, cream, milk, cheeses, coconut oil and palm oil. Mono- and polyunsaturated fat are found mainly in fish (such as salmon and trout) and also in seeds, avocados and plant oils (for instance olive oil and sunflower oil). Trans fats (also known as trans-fatty acids or TFAs) occur in small amounts in various animal products, and are formed when vegetable oils are put through the hydrogenation process to make margarine, shortening, and cooking oils for use in processed foods such as cookies, fried foods, and cakes. TFAs are used by manufacturers as they allow foods to have a longer shelf life and give food desirable shape, taste, and texture.

To reduce total, saturated and TFA fats, use low-fat versions of dairy products (such as semi-skim or skim milk), buy lean cuts of meat, remove visible fat, and skin from the meat before you cook it, and use less fat in cooking (broil and bake rather than fry or roast). Choose small amounts of fats and oils that are rich in monounsaturates (e.g., olive oil) or polyunsaturates (e.g., sunflower oil) rather than saturated fats such as butter.

How to get the right fat in your diet

Keep in mind the advice from the American Heart Association:

- Fat should account for less than 25 to 35 percent of your total calorie intake each day.
- Most fat in your diet should be unsaturated.
- Less than 7 percent of calories should be from saturated fat.
- Less than 1 percent of calories should be from trans fats.
- You should limit your cholesterol intake to less than 300 milligrams per day (less than 200 milligrams per day if you have heart disease)
- Beware the fat hidden in packaged and processed foods—always check labels. Avoid trans fats, and remember that unhydrogenated vegetable oils are better than hydrogenated ones.
- Choose soft margarine instead of butter.

LEARN TO BE IDLE

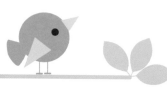

Apart from being pleasurable, doing nothing in a mindful way is an excellent way to enhance wellbeing. When we replace scattered thoughts with focused attention, the calming effects can be transformative.

Mindfulness and particularly meditation, have been scientifically proven to reduce stress, improve memory, and enhance creativity and overall feelings of wellbeing. The more you practice, the easier it becomes to enjoy the benefits of a calm, focused mind. An easy way to begin is to sit in nature and contemplate a beautiful scene. The simple act of looking at a single bloom in your garden for a minute or two can produce a profound feeling of calm and relaxation. So put away the to-do lists, shut down technology, find a quiet spot, and just be.

Here's a simple 10-minute exercise to practice resting the mind:

- Sit or lie in a comfortable position in a quiet place where you won't be disturbed for 10 minutes or so.
- Quiet your thoughts and take a few deep breaths in and out, concentrating on the sound of your breathing and the flow of air through your nostrils.
- If unwanted thoughts come up, observe them briefly, then go back to the breathing and let them pass.
- Remain like this for around 10 minutes, or longer if possible.
- Gently refocus on your surroundings and enjoy the sense of calm you have achieved.

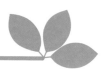

LOVE LIKE A BUDDHA

Loving-kindness is a form of Buddhist meditation that aims to develop altruistic love while healing troubled minds. First you must learn to love yourself. Then you can direct feelings of loving-kindness towards four chosen individuals: A figure of respect, such as a spiritual teacher; a close family member or friend; a neutral person; and a hostile person.

According to Buddhist teaching, if you send loving-kindness from person to person in the above order, it will break down the barriers between the four people and yourself—and the effect will be to break down the divisions within your own mind. Visualize each person in turn and reflect on their positive qualities. Then make a positive statement about that person in your own words. Follow this by repeating an internalized mantra or phrase such as "loving-kindness."

FIRST YOU MUST LEARN TO LOVE YOURSELF. THEN YOU CAN DIRECT FEELINGS OF LOVING-KINDNESS TO OTHERS.

91

CHECK YOUR RISKS

The degree to which diabetes can shorten life depends on a variety of factors, including the type of diabetes (whether it is Type 1 insulin-dependent diabetes, which tends to be more severe, or Type 2, which tends to be associated with adult onset and obesity), the age at which it is diagnosed and whether you have other risk factors that add complications, such as heart disease. Poorly controlled diabetes could take five years from your average life expectancy.

In diabetes the body is unable to move sugar from the blood into the cells because of inadequate insulin supplies. Blood sugar levels rise while the cells must use alternative sources of energy. This wreaks havoc on the blood vessels, including the coronary arteries supplying the heart. As many as 75 percent of people with diabetes develop cardiovascular disease as well. Diabetes also damages the nerves and can cause kidney failure and blindness. It leads to an increased susceptibility to infection and impaired immune function as well, leaving you less able to fight other diseases.

Diabetes: Know the risks

- Besides age and weight, what factors increase your risk for Type 2 diabetes?

  - If you have a parent, brother, or sister with diabetes.

  - If your family background is Alaska Native, American Indian, Afro-Caribbean, African, South Asian (Indian, Pakistani), Pacific islander, Hispanic/Latino.

  - If you have had gestational diabetes, or have given birth to at least one baby weighing more than 9 pounds.

  - If your blood pressure is 140/90 mm Hg or higher, or you have been told that you have high blood pressure.

  - If your cholesterol levels are not normal. Your HDL cholesterol ("good" cholesterol) is below 35 mg/dL (0.9 mmol/L), or your triglyceride level is above 250 mg/dL (2.8 mmol/L).

  - If you are fairly inactive, exercising fewer than three times a week.

  - If you have polycystic ovary syndrome, also called PCOS (women only).

  - If you've had impaired glucose tolerance (IGT) or impaired fasting glucose (IFG).

  - If you have other clinical conditions associated with insulin resistance, such as *acanthosis nigricans*.

  - If you have a history of cardiovascular disease.

- Recognize the symptoms. These include increased thirst, passing urine more frequently, weight loss, tiredness, blurred vision, hunger, and increased infections.

- Get diagnosed early. As many as one in three are unaware they have the condition, while high blood-sugar levels silently damage their tissues.

- Control your weight. If you are at high risk of developing diabetes, a 7 percent weight loss and 150 minutes of moderate-intensity exercise each week will halve that risk. Once diabetes is established, losing weight may help you to live longer. Researchers at the University of Surrey, UK, found that obesity in diabetics can reduce life expectancy by eight years.

GO FOR GARLIC

Garlic has been used all over the world as both food and medicine for thousands of years. Scientific studies suggest that this humble bulb has many therapeutic benefits—it can help to reduce the risk of developing lung cancer, lower the risk of osteoarthritis and protect the heart from damage.

Consuming garlic regularly can prevent infections of all kinds and even reduce the risk of catching the common cold. It can also be used to detoxify the body, as it has sulfur-containing compounds that activate the liver enzymes responsible for expelling toxins.

Summer is garlic season and with its pungent, creamy flavor, it's a delicious way to pack more nutrients into your meals.

Try these simple recipes using raw and cooked garlic (raw is best):
- Purée fresh garlic with cannellini beans, tahini, olive oil, and lemon juice to make a healthy dip.
- Add garlic and fresh lemon juice to steamed spinach or other steamed vegetables.
- Roast whole garlic cloves, chop, and add them to a creamy pasta salad.
- Combine parsley, citrus, or mint with garlic to help sweeten the breath.

COMFORTABLE CLIMATE

The climate around us greatly influences many aspects of health and disease. At its extremes, cold weather brings the threat of exposure, hypothermia, and infections such as influenza, bronchitis, and pneumonia, while excessively hot weather can put intolerable strain on the heart and cause problems with dehydration. The very old and very young are most vulnerable, especially when seasonal tolls such as influenza epidemics strike.

Somewhere between these is the ideal climate, where the winters are mild and the summers are pleasantly warm. Sardinia may just represent the perfect spot. A remarkably high proportion of people who live there reach their hundredth year, including, unusually, a large number of men—there are 13.56 centenarians per 100,000 people in this balmy region. Or try Okinawa in Japan, where the temperature hovers around and above 68°F (20°C) for most of the year and, astonishingly, more than 40 out of 100,000 people are over 100 years old. The critical aspect in these places seems to be that many of those who reach the age of 80 proceed to survive for much longer—this is the stage at which we are most sensitive to the effects of climate and least able to cope with harsh conditions. Pack your bags now!

ONE WAY TICKET

BOOST YOUR ANTIOXIDANTS

One of the main theories about why the body degenerates as we age is based on a chemical process called oxidation. During normal metabolism, the body produces unstable molecules called free radicals. Other factors in the environment around us also increase free-radical production. Free radicals cause oxidation—this is dangerous as it damages the body's cells and tissues, and has been implicated in all the major killer diseases.

Fortunately, we have a supply of natural antidotes called antioxidants, which mop up free radicals. But levels of antioxidants fall as we age, leading to increasing damage to cells and tissues. By increasing our intake of antioxidants as we get older (or avoiding free-radical-producing pollutants), we may be able to protect ourselves from this process.

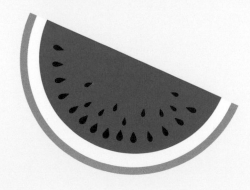

A WIDE RANGE OF CHEMICALS FOUND IN DIFFERENT FOODS CAN ACT AS ANTIOXIDANTS, SO KEEP YOUR DIET HEALTHY AND VARIED.

A wide range of chemicals found in different foods can act as antioxidants, but some of the most important are beta-carotene and the antioxidant vitamins A, C, and E. As far as antioxidant supplements go, however, studies have been disappointing. Some trials found only minimal and inconsistent evidence that any single vitamin supplement, combined antioxidant supplement, or multivitamin combination has a significant benefit in cardiovascular disease, while others found that beta-carotene used to prevent cancer might even increase the risk of death from other causes. Research on people who follow a diet rich in antioxidants, rather than relying on supplements, however, has been promising, for example in reducing the risk of Alzheimer's disease. Something in the chemical complexity of food could be key here. The best advice for now is simply to keep your diet healthy and varied.

Foods that are rich in antioxidants:

Beans: pinto, red, black, and kidney beans

Berries: cranberries, blueberries, and blackberries

Nuts: pecans, walnuts, and hazelnuts

Other fruits: plums, cherries, apples

Artichoke hearts

Russet potatoes

95

VISIT THE LIBRARY

Of course, we're not going to stop reading books, but you don't have to buy them all. Book manufacture, like almost all industries, takes energy, electricity, and fossil fuel burning power that emits carbon dioxide and other greenhouse gases. Each book takes many processes to bring it to publication—the receipt and editing of manuscripts, which involves computers and printers, heating and air conditioning, lighting, pens and paper, and telephones. Turning those manu- scripts into the pages of a book involves chopping down trees, debarking the wood, and pulping it for the printers. Each of these stages requires energy and emissions to transport the materials, whether ferrying the wood, the pulp, paper, or the books themselves to storage warehouses and bookshops. Taken together, all these stages add up, totaling about 5.5 lbs (2.5 kg) of CO_2 per paperback, according to Penguin Books.

So for book junkies, there are a number of ways to feed an addiction while reducing your carbon footprint. Libraries are a good place to start, as is sharing books among friends. Secondhand shops are a great idea for reducing your carbon footprint, and are usually cheaper than buying brand new. You can browse secondhand bookshops from the comfort of your own home via the Internet; for example, Abebooks is similar to eBay and brings together 13,500 used book sellers from around the world.

THINK YOUNG

Thinking young is one of the simplest ways to boost your well-being, whatever your age. You don't have to squeeze yourself into the latest dance gear or save up for cosmetic surgery—just keep an open mind to life's endless possibilities.

Relish new challenges, learn new skills, and set new goals. Embrace new technology, and use what you need from it. Scorn convention—if there is something that you really want to do then find a way to do it. Never utter the words "I'm too old" (sometimes this might be true, but just don't dwell on it!). Why talk about your age? Once you're over 18 no one needs to know it.

In keeping with the trend for women living longer than men, the oldest person ever is a woman. Jeanne-Louise Calment holds the Guinness World Record, having lived 122 years and 164 days. She was born in France in 1875 and she died in 1997. She was already 14 when the Eiffel Tower in Paris was completed in 1889 and was still riding a bicycle at 100. At the age of 114 she portrayed herself in the film *Vincent and Me*, in order to become the oldest actress in film.

TRY A MEDITERRANEAN DIET

It's not just the sun and sea they're blessed with. Scientific research has shown that people who live in the Mediterranean are the best candidates for longevity, and enjoy low rates of heart disease. Their life-prolonging diet is linked to a lower death rate from all sorts of diseases, including heart disease, and may also reduce the risk of Alzheimer's by as much as 40 percent.

Key to this diet is the generous amount of fruit, vegetables, and nuts consumed, and the lack of processed foods. Increasing fruit and vegetables from two to five portions a day can greatly reduce the risk of many cancers, while it's also known that a vegetarian diet is linked to a premature death rate 20 percent lower than for meat eaters.

But it's the whole lifestyle that counts: Also central to this culture are two other factors you can't ignore—more physical activity, and an extended social support system.

What to have in your pantry
Although there is great diversity between Mediterranean countries, common dietary threads include large amounts of fruit, vegetables, beans, nuts, cereals, and seeds; olive oil, fish, and poultry consumed in moderation; a little red meat and dairy produce; and wine, but again, drunk in moderation.

GET CREATIVE

Close links exist between creativity and happiness. Among the therapeutic benefits of creative activity are enhanced focus greater self-esteem, a sense of control over one's life, and increased energy and contentment.

Creative activities can also help to reduce your risk of memory loss as you grow older. Scientists from the Mayo Clinic studied 197 people between the ages of 70 and 89 who had signs of either mild cognitive impairment or memory loss. They compared them with another 1,124 people in the same age bracket who had no signs of memory problems. Researchers concluded that people who had participated in crafts or other such activities during that period of their life were 40 percent less likely to develop memory loss than those who had not. Undertaking and persevering with projects in knitting, quilting, and pottery is believed to be especially beneficial.

PURIFY WITH PLANTS

Colorful plants can brighten your mood as well as your surroundings, not to mention help the environment. Wildflower gardens are ideal, since they mainly consist of either indigenous species or plants that are well-suited to the local weather conditions. Getting them growing initially tends to take just as much work as any other garden, but once the wildflowers have begun to flourish, they will provide food and sanctuary for local wildlife like butterflies, songbirds, toads, and other creatures.

If you live in a drier climate, there are lots of species that need very little water, and they don't all look spindly or desert-like. You don't have to go for cacti, pines, or small hairy succulents with narrow, tiny leaves if these aren't to your taste. Verdant plants and delicate flowers such as juniper, nasturtiums, sage, iris, thyme, crocus, lavender, evening primrose, yucca gloriosa, california poppy, gold dust, and many others all do well in dry, sunny conditions.

POLISH YOUR HALO

Low self-esteem can gnaw away at life. People with higher levels of self-esteem value themselves more, and so put more effort into looking after their health and well-being. They also tend to be happier people.

There are positive steps you can take to build up your self-esteem if it is at a low ebb. Start by making a list of your good points, and don't be hard on yourself. Once you have your list, it is important to abandon modesty and congratulate yourself frequently on these points every day.

Another great way to boost your self-image is to learn a new skill—origami, playing the saxophone, skydiving—it really doesn't matter what you choose, but take it seriously and practice it until you can do it well in order to get the most benefit from it.

Doing something nice for others has been shown to increase our self-esteem— find a community group you can volunteer with, preferably one that interests you. The chance to polish your halo on a regular basis by helping others is one of the most powerful ways to build self-esteem.

WHAT'S STOPPING YOU?

We hope this book has inspired you and left you feeling optimistic that it is possible to take your fitness and wellbeing into your own hands. You should now have a better understanding of the positive steps you can take toward achieving a long and fulfilled life, one that is mindful of others, and of the world around you.

You should also have gained a sense of the effort that is sometimes involved in adopting a healthier way of life. Many of the easy options in life are the least healthy choices, and you may have to start asking yourself questions about what needs to change if you are to achieve your lifestyle goals. In order to truly live well, it's usually necessary to look beyond the quick rewards and invest in a way of life that slowly brings longer-term benefits to yourself, and to others. But, having read this book, you are perfectly equipped with 100 ways to wellness to help you make this journey one step at a time.

Along the way you're going to need some good help, support, and information, so listen closely to the comments and advice of those around you. Think carefully about what your friends, family, or colleagues say, and remember that, when it comes to health, most advice must be weighed up in the context of any individual's own life and medical background. Beware hype—double-check specific medical information by playing detective in the library or on the Internet. Use your common sense and instincts to sift opinion from fact, then work out what might be right for you—it's time to start taking your first steps toward living well!

INDEX

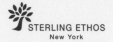

STERLING ETHOS
New York

An Imprint of Sterling Publishing Co., Inc.
1166 Avenue of the Americas
New York, NY 10036

Conceived and produced by
Elwin Street Limited
14 Clerkenwell Green
London EC1R 0DP
www.elwinstreet.com

ISBN 978-1-4549-3567-4

Distributed in Canada by Sterling Publishing Co., Inc.
c/o Canadian Manda Group, 664 Annette Street
Toronto, Ontario M6S 2C8, Canada

For information about custom editions, special sales, and premium and corporate purchases, please contact Sterling Special Sales at 800-805-5489 or specialsales@sterlingpublishing.com.

Manufactured in China

2 4 6 8 10 9 7 5 3 1

www.sterlingpublishing.com

Designed and illustrated by Karin Skånberg

Disclaimer: The advice, recipes and exercises in this book are intended as a personal guide to healthy living. However, this information is not intended to provide medical advice and it should not replace the guidance of a qualified physician or other healthcare professional. Decisions about your health should be made by you and your healthcare provider based on the specific circumstances of your health, risk factors, family history and other considerations. See your healthcare provider before making major dietary changes or embarking on an exercise programme, especially if you have existing health problems, medical conditions or chronic diseases. The author and publishers have made every effort to ensure that the information in this book is safe and accurate, but they cannot accept liability for any resulting injury or loss or damage to either property or person, whether direct or consequential and howsoever arising.

The information in this study is based on thorough academic research, with information gathered from over 100 journal articles, and informed by book-length studies, case studies, reports and statistics. For a full list of references, please contact the publisher.